Calisthenics

by Mark Lauren & Joshua Clark

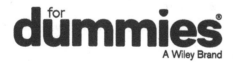

A Wiley Brand

Calisthenics For Dummies®

Published by: **John Wiley & Sons, Inc.,** 111 River Street, Hoboken, NJ 07030-5774, www.wiley.com

Copyright © 2024 by John Wiley & Sons, Inc., Hoboken, New Jersey

Media and software compilation copyright © 2024 by John Wiley & Sons, Inc. All rights reserved.

Published simultaneously in Canada

For general information on our other products and services, please contact our Customer Care Department within the US at 877-762-2974, outside the US at 317-572-3993, or fax 317-572-4002. For technical support, please visit https://hub.wiley.com/community/support/dummies.

Wiley publishes in a variety of print and electronic formats and by print-on-demand. Some material included with standard print versions of this book may not be included in e-books or in print-on-demand. If this book refers to media such as a CD or DVD that is not included in the version you purchased, you may download this material at http://booksupport.wiley.com. For more information about Wiley products, visit www.wiley.com.

Library of Congress Control Number: 2023949846

ISBN 978-1-394-19611-1 (pbk); ISBN 978-1-394-19613-5 (ePDF); ISBN 978-1-394-19612-8 (epub)

SKY10081720_080924

Table of Contents

Introduction

Welcome to *Calisthenics For Dummies,* your guide on the journey to your best body through the most functional form of fitness.

About This Book

This book is intended to be one-stop fitness shopping. It can become the only equipment you ever need to work out your entire body again, quickly and effectively.

Whether you're an elite athlete or someone who hasn't exercised in decades, whether you're 18 or 80, you'll discover all you need to form your fitness foundation and build your peak physique in this book.

We teach you to rebrand athleticism by dissecting its secrets. We show you how calisthenics doesn't train you for a specific sport — it trains you for life. Each workout helps prepare you for the muscular, joint, bone, and even mental stresses of life. That's what real fitness does. The fitter you become, the more you can move through life with ease.

This book walks you step by step through a lifelong bodyweight exercise program and addresses some special needs people have, such as working out with limited mobility.

The most important takeaway from this book is proper joint alignment. You'll find tips and techniques peppered throughout the book to help you achieve this, because it is the only way to reach your own personal pinnacle of fitness, safely, for now and for the rest of your life.

Conventions Used in This Book

We've established the following conventions to make it easier for you to navigate this book:

>> New terms are in *italics,* and we define them for you.

>> **Bold** text highlights key words in bulleted lists and action parts in numbered lists.

>> Monofont sets off web addresses.

Foolish Assumptions

In writing this book, we've made some assumptions about you:

>> You may be afraid that working out is going to be too tough, take up too much of your time, or be a drudgery (it's not!).

>> Whether you consider yourself fit or not, there's probably some key elements missing from your fitness foundation. Without a strong foundation, whatever body you build is going to be more fragile and prone to injury than it should be.

How This Book Is Organized

This book begins by helping you feel comfortable with calisthenics, and progresses into teaching you exactly what you need to reach your individual goals.

To make the content more accessible, we divided it into five parts:

Part 1: Total Fitness, No Limits includes three chapters that explain why calisthenics are the most effective and efficient method of exercise for everyone, the secrets to attaining your best body, and how to say motivated.

Part 2: The Exercises includes seven chapters of over one hundred exercises covering floor routines, developmental movements, and strength training exercises for your core, legs, chest, shoulders, triceps, back, biceps, and forearms.

Part 3: The Workouts includes two chapters designed to help you set goals, including and a 13-week program you can modify to your ends.

Part 4: Calisthenics for Special Circumstances includes four chapters covering nine-minute workouts, how to work out when you're pregnant or have limited mobility, and also how to help your kids get excited about fitness.

Part 5: The Part of Tens includes two chapters that give you a buffet of tips to tone and tighten and how to be successful, as well as a chapter that debunks the top ten bodyweight training myths.

Icons Used in This Book

In the margins of almost every page of this book, you find icons, which are there to alert you to different types of information. Here's what they mean:

TIP

This icon saves you time and energy by showing you a helpful method for doing something.

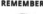

REMEMBER

This icon points out important information you need to know as you develop your drawing skills.

WARNING

This icon points out potential problems and positive solutions.

Beyond the Book

In addition to the book content, you can find valuable free material online. We provide you with a Cheat Sheet that serves as a quick checklist, including information about the performance pyramid, how to be successful, how to work on your technique and posture, and more. Check out this book's online Cheat Sheet by searching www.dummies.com for **Calisthenics for Dummies Cheat Sheet**.

Where to Go from Here

Although everyone can gain something from every section of this book, Parts 1–3 contain the exercises you need for lifelong fitness success. It's important to note that virtually everyone can benefit from not only the exercises and workouts themselves, but from understanding the secrets to moving through life like an athlete.

Feel free to skip over chapters in Part 4 if none of those special circumstances apply to you, although an unfortunate reality is that most of us will face limited mobility from a (hopefully minor) injury at some point. Part 5 is intended to help build your fitness wisdom. After all, it's difficult to do something effectively without understanding why you're doing it.

1
Total Fitness: No Limits

Discovering why calisthenics is the most effective and efficient method of exercise for all bodies and abilities.

Learning the secrets to attaining your best body and moving it through life with ease.

Setting specific goals, staying motivated, and overcoming obstacles that stand in the way of success.

Chapter **1**

Calisthenics: When Your Body Is Your Equipment

Congratulations! You're now holding the only thing you need — other than your own body — to get into the best shape of your life.

We've already done the hard work for you: Distilling three decades of experience and a billion-dollars-worth of complex sports science down to a simple, lifelong program that takes less than 1 percent of your time each week.

The exercises in this book comprehensively and methodically cover all muscle groups, joint functions, and athletic skills. And they're for people of all abilities. They can help you get and stay strong, lean, healthy, mobile, and injury free.

Calisthenics: For All Bodies and Abilities

With calisthenics and bodyweight exercises, you use the body you have to build the body you want. You don't even need to use equipment or machines. You were born with world's most advanced fitness machine: You.

What's so great about this fitness machine is that it's always there. It is the one and only thing you are never without. It's no longer necessary to spend hours at a gym. In fact, you don't have to go to a gym at all.

With these workouts you will not waste a single moment of your valued time using ineffective training methods. And no longer will you be able to use the #1 excuse for not training: "I don't have the time."

Because bodyweight movements are the safest and most functional exercises, they are for people of *all* athletic ability levels. The ones in this book are tailored to suit many needs and lifestyles. Clear, concise, and complete, we bring these exercises into your home, workplace, nearby park, or wherever you like.

REMEMBER

The metric of your merit is not based on the amount of weight you can lift. Instead, it's all about performance. Gauge your success by how properly you can perform an exercise. This is the most fundamental idea of calisthenics.

Posture and ideal joint alignment determine performance in all you do. Proper performance, as you'll soon see, determines your athletic skills, and in turn, your appearance. At the end of the day, we all want to look good.

Why Calisthenics Is Better than Any Other Workout

This section outlines the top eight advantages that calisthenics has over working out with equipment. These are the reasons so many people who start a bodyweight program actually stick with it.

You save time

Let's do some quick math. Say it takes you 25 minutes each way to get to and from the gym, and then another 45 minutes to use a bunch of machines. That's one and a half hours per workout. Do that three times a week, and you're at four and half hours. That's over half of a work day. Who wants to sacrifice that amount of time?

With calisthenics, there's no packing, traveling, parking, or changing at the gym, then doing it all in reverse to get back home.

Also, trying to work out your whole body by exercising muscle groups separately, with machines and dumbbells that isolate only certain muscles, is unfunctional and inefficient. It takes far less time to get a full body workout when you're actually doing full body exercises.

You save money

Instead of fancy fitness contraptions, gym memberships, parking, and gallons of gas, for just the price of this book, you now have a lifelong fitness program.

You save space

You only need to temporarily create enough space to lie down in. And there's no need to store whatever latest contraptions are gathering dust in your home.

You can do it anywhere

You can turn any area into your fitness center: Your bedroom, living room, garage, driveway, yard, office, park, playground, beach — you name it. And if you're traveling, there's no need to search for the nearest gym. You can turn your hotel room, just like almost any other place on Earth, into a full fitness center.

No gymbarrassment

Plenty of folks want to get in shape, but cringe at the thought of putting themselves on display at a fitness center. But with bodyweight exercises, you are the boss now: Crank those tunes up as loud as you please or watch whatever channel you want. No gym clothes required. (In fact, no clothes at all are required.)

It's always open

Early in the morning, late at night, Christmas, New Year's, snowstorms — you name it. You can work out wherever and whenever it fits your busy schedule.

It's safer

Many people who try aerobics hurt themselves, even when it's "low-impact." By using motions that are natural for your body, these low impact bodyweight exercises help you avoid the myriad chronic and acute injuries like joint problems associated with weight lifting. Of course, you should always consult a qualified doctor before beginning any fitness program.

You will not stop seeing results

This is not some short-term fix or fad, but a fun, functional program that will never stop working for you. Variety is the spice of life. This book provides many ways to vary these exercises so you won't get stuck in a rut. Instead they'll remain enjoyable and they never stop increasing your fitness. Keeping your muscles guessing is how you keep them growing.

Getting the Results You Want

For thousands of years — from Ancient Greece's Olympic athletes to tomorrow's Special Operations forces — humanity's greatest physical specimens have *not* relied on fitness centers in their towns or dumbbells in their homes. Instead they mastered the art of moving around what matters most: their own bodies.

Become stronger

Rarely do you do anything in life that isolates only a single muscle group. Our bodies were designed to become stronger as a whole. It's how you not only look your best, but feel your best.

But most weight training exercises only isolate certain muscles, requiring a fairly small portion of your body's total muscle mass. In contrast, even the most focused bodyweight exercises not only emphasize your "targeted" muscle groups, but, unlike using those fancy machines in the gym, they develop your stabilizer muscles that surround the targeted area as well, and do a far better job of that than using free weights either. This creates more muscle, and more muscle means burning more fat!

Burn more fat

These exercises will crank your body's metabolism better than using weights or aerobics, because they build more muscle. And muscle is the most metabolically expensive tissue we can manipulate, meaning it burns up a lot of calories — even at rest.

This is a prime example of the snowball effect: The more muscle you have, the more calories you burn, and so the less you have to worry about what you eat. While the less muscle you have, the more likely it is that extra calories will turn into fat. And so you're more prone to become overweight, and get stuck in a never-ending battle of guilt vs. goodies when it comes to food.

Get better with age

It takes about ten calories a day just to keep one pound of muscle alive, even if you are completely inactive. An extra five pounds of muscle can burn up to 1,500 calories in a month — that's the equivalent of five pounds of fat per year, which more than reverses some negative effects of aging on your metabolism.

Regain your youthful metabolism

One reason many people gain weight as they age, especially beginning in their 30s, is because they have less muscle than they had in their late teens and early twenties. As we age, our bodies naturally lose muscle, especially if we become less active. This muscle tissue loss results in a decreasing metabolic rate. And then, if you continue to eat like you did when you were younger . . . Well, you'll slowly gain weight, pound by pound, month by month, year by year, until one day you look in the mirror and wonder, "What happened?" This is how the average American adult gains 2.2 pounds per year.

The key to eliminating accumulated body fat is regaining your youthful metabolism by regaining your muscle through strength training.

Live injury free

Most aerobic activities carry with them a great risk of injury. Even so-called "low impact" classes or activities like stationary cycling are not necessarily low-impact. Things like running are extremely high-impact, damaging to your knees, hips and back. Aerobic dance is even worse.

Sure, you'll hear the occasional genetic exception declare that they've never been injured doing these exercises. But overuse injuries are cumulative and often build undetected over years until it's too late, leading to a decrease or loss of mobility as you age, which, in turn, too often leads to a shortened lifespan.

In contrast, the movements in this book, when done properly, have virtually zero impact. You'll be moving your body how it was designed to move. Not how it gets broken.

Getting Comfortable with Bodyweight Exercises

To beginners, it can feel pretty weird trying to exercise without the typical exercise machines. Instead, you're going to start using your body the way it was meant to be used — the way you used it when you were first learning to crawl, walk, run, and climb.

Use muscles you didn't know you had

With the proper bodyweight movements, you can isolate and work all your muscles. Everything from your neck to toes are fair game and tied together. You'll discover muscles you have and muscles that might that have atrophied in our modern sedentary lifestyles. You will literally become a stronger person.

Get off the bench

Your arms were made to push and pull your bodyweight, not to grasp handles on machines or metal bars while you sit on a bench. I mean, lying down on a soft surface is just fine — when you're sleeping. Sitting on a cushioned seat is fine if you're driving, or looking at your computer or TV. But not if you're doing real exercise.

Discovering the Eight Abilities You'll Build Through Calisthenics

We realize most people are reading this book because they want to look and feel better, not necessarily improve their balance, flexibility, and coordination. But this is a common misconception and many programs put the cart before the horse. By focusing on developing these eight skills, you will make your best gains, both in ability and in appearance.

In the decade I spent honing military units assigned to carry out the most dangerous missions, it was always my experience that the individual with the best development in all areas of physical ability succeeds the best operationally.

This program develops the entire spectrum of physical skills. Form follows function. You look your healthiest by being your healthiest. Your physique and your fitness are determined by the degree to which you possess the following eight qualities that define fitness.

Muscular strength

Your ability to exert a force through a given distance, muscular strength can be determined by the difficulty of an exercise that you are able to perform for a single repetition. For example, if Tarzan, with maximal effort, can perform one normal push-up but Jane can perform a handstand push-up, then Jane has greater muscular strength.

Power

Power is the amount of force you can exert in a specific amount of time. Power = Work/Time. If Tarzan and Jane are both able to perform one pull-up with maximal effort, but Jane can perform that one pull-up faster, then she has more power even though they have the same strength.

Muscular endurance

Muscular endurance is how long you can exert a specific force. Jane and Tarzan could compare their muscular endurance by seeing who can hold the peak position of the pull-up the longest.

Cardiovascular endurance

This is your body's ability to supply working muscles with oxygen during prolonged activity. Jane and Tarzan challenge and improve their cardiovascular endurance by performing 200 non-stop squats together.

Speed

Speed is measured as your ability to rapidly and repeatedly execute a movement or a series of movements. If Jane can do 45 lunges in 30 seconds and Tarzan can do 25, then Jane has greater speed.

Coordination

Coordination is your ability to combine more than one movement to create a single, distinct movement. For example, performing a simple jump requires that you coordinate several movements. The bend at the waist, knees, and ankles and then the correct extension of those joints must all be combined into a single movement. Your ability to combine these movements, with the proper timing, into one movement determines your coordination, and in turn, how well you can do the exercise.

Balance

Balance is your ability to maintain control of your body's center of gravity.

Flexibility

Flexibility is your range of motion. If Jane, while doing a squat and using good form, can go down until her bottom touches her heels, and Tarzan can only go until his thighs are parallel to the ground, then Jane has greater flexibility.

Rounding Up Your Gear for Home Workouts

As you've seen, you don't need equipment to achieve optimal fitness. But some readers might prefer to complement a calisthenics program with movements — such as isolation exercises — that involve equipment, perhaps to focus on particular muscle groups to meet their particular goals.

You'd be surprised at how much resistance equipment you can create from basic household items, replacing the need for dumbbells in traditional strength exercises.

Take bicep curls for example. Just because you don't have dumbbells doesn't mean you can't do them. You can use gallon jugs of water (filled to your appropriate level), grocery bags filled with things, big books, bricks, soup cans, or my favorite whether I'm at home or in another country: a backpack. Check out Figure 1-1 for examples of the gear discussed in the following sections.

A backpack

You can fill a backpack (or duffel bag) with books, magazines, newspapers, cans of food, rocks, sand, and/or full water bottles. Add to the backpack until you have the perfect weight and hold the top strap. You can even make a proper handle out of it: Just break off a few inches of a stick or branch that's the proper width for a handle and use tape to fasten it to the backpack's top handle. Most backpacks can easily hold up to 60 pounds, some a lot more.

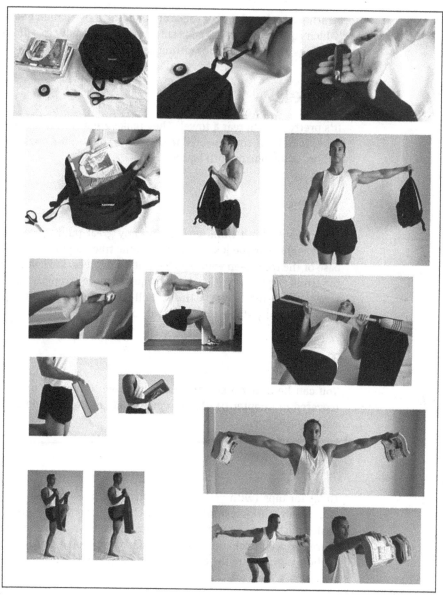

FIGURE 1-1: Calisthenics involves simple body weight exercises you can do in your home with normal, everyday objects.

© John Wiley & Sons

You can use backpacks in place of dumbbells for myriad movements like bicep curls, shoulder raises, tricep exercises, and upright rows. Throw it on your back to increase the resistance to any pull-up, squat, lunge — you name it. (Or give your child a piggyback during leg exercises.)

Wearing a backpack full of rocks and holding a five gallon bucket filled with water (which equals 40 pounds) adds some serious intensity to calf raises. You can place sandbags on your knees for sitting calf raises.

Towels

It's pretty hard to tear a towel. They make great makeshift straps (as do ropes or belts) for let-me-ins (covered in Chapter 9) by looping one around a tree, fence or railing, using one or both hands.

Trees

Some people don't think you can do any great pulling exercises with only your bodyweight. But you just need to try some tree-hugging. Put your feet around the base of the tree, keep your legs bent at 90 degrees, stick your butt out, grab on to the trunk (higher is easier, lower requires more strength) and you can crank out some let-me-ins — maybe the best all-around pulling exercise there is. Likewise, you can use any stable railing or pole or post.

Table

You can lie under a strong desk or kitchen table and use it to do let-me-ups (covered in Chapter 9). Or put your hands on top and do triceps extensions, or easier push-ups.

Chairs

Great for dips (with your legs out straight, heels on the floor or up on another chair) and triceps extensions. Two chairs also create a great raised surface for easier push-ups. You can bring your chest down into the empty space between them for deep push-ups. And put your feet up on a third chair or surface — the higher your feet are the more intense the push-up.

Video camera

It's a superb idea to film yourself doing new movements. That way, you can see what you're doing wrong and how to do it better. Remember, posture = performance = results.

Pull-up bar

Relatively inexpensive and easy to install, these bars can be used for any kind of pull-up you can imagine. Or install them at waist height for triceps extensions, let me ups, and let me ins.

Bosu ball

A Bosu ball creates an unstable surface to put any of your limbs on. Unstable surfaces require more core strength because they utilize your stabilizer muscles.

Try putting one hand on a basketball for push-ups. If you're really advanced, you can roll the basketball back and forth between hands between reps.

You can also try one-legged leg exercises on a pillow. Unstable surface forces your muscles (and your all-important stabilizer muscles) to work harder. Just be aware of maintaining your balance so to avoid injury.

Suspension straps

Suspension straps give you the ability to alter the height of your hands or legs to your liking. Plus, they have the added ability of being unstable, thus requiring more of your muscles and joints.

Elastic bands

Elastic bands are much easier on your joints than weights. They come in different strengths, and you can even stack them together and attach a few at once to the handles to really increase the resistance.

You can put them around trees, railings, poles, fences, or underfoot. The best way to make these truly versatile is to screw strong hooks into a vertical post (like a 4x4 or wall stud) at different heights and use these as anchors. Then there's just about no upper body exercise you can't do with elastic bands.

WHAT TO WEAR, WHAT TO WEAR

TIP

The great thing about working out in privacy is that you can wear anything at all. Including nothing. Of course, if you do wear clothes (an especially good idea in public!), be sure they are baggy or flexible enough that they don't constrict your movements. Since you're moving how nature intended, bare feet are fine. Or else some light shoes with very basic support, like Keds, are great.

Since you're not doing high impact activities that put a lot of stress on your feet, you don't need expensive sport shoes or thick insoles. Often, shoes with thick, soft soles are a detriment for your legs, because they can cause your stabilizer muscles to disengage since there's less risk of strong impact with the ground. Ideally, the muscles in your feet, ankles, and calves are stabilizing and supporting you. Not your insoles.

Your Body Is Your Home

Your real home is not your apartment or your house or your city or even your country, but your *body*. It is the only thing you, your heart, your soul, and your mind, will always live inside as long as you walk the earth. It is the single most important physical thing in this world that you can take care of.

We all have a choice: To take care of ourselves or to simply let time takes its toll. If you truly want to look and feel better, you have everything you need to do that, right now. The good news is that taking care of your body is mentally and physically uplifting. In addition to controlling your waistline and increasing your energy, exercise can clear your mind and reduce stress. Also, it just really feels good to take care of yourself.

TIP

A realistic goal for fitness requires an understanding of nutritional basics, as well as working out 20-30 minutes a day, 4-5 times a week — that's about 1 percent of your time. That's all you really need.

Adding exercise to your life can help you meet life's obstacles with physical, mental, and spiritual strength. You'll thrive on the energy exercise gives you every day. It can mitigate many of the bad things in life — depression, anxiety, nervousness, tension, boredom, and impatience. It can help you think more clearly. It can help you stay mobile as you age. Remember that only you are in control of how you treat your body. Don't let the excuses hijack your journey to a healthy mind and body. You've taken the first step by buying this book. Let's get started!

Chapter **2**

You Were Made to Move

No matter your age, ability, or body type, you probably picked this book up because you want to get into better shape. You want to *look* better and *feel* better. Thankfully, those two goals are one and the same.

But why do so many fitness programs fail to achieve them? One reason is because they fail to define what fitness actually means. This chapter talks about why getting and staying active is so critical to your health and well-being and then covers some body kinetics that will help you understand how your body functions best.

Fitness Equals Function

What kind of body do you want? One that moves through this physical world with ease and efficiency? People typically find the most *capable* body the most beautiful. A few decades of industry and technology haven't undone a hundred millennia — humans are still programmed to desire being, and being with, the people who can find food and defend them. Those who not only survive but protect and take care of them.

Practice the movements most important to your survival

When you gain strength through highly functional training, your body displays your self-mastery, which leads to mastery of your environment, and that is exactly what humans need to survive and reproduce.

Put the pieces together

After decades of research, writing, and training, I amassed all the pieces to the giant fitness puzzle. But it remained just that: in pieces. One big, needlessly complicated mess.

No one seemed able to distill the essence of what it truly takes to become strong and lean into something simple yet comprehensive. So I went back to how I planned missions in the military.

I started with the objective, then worked backward to find the most efficient strategy to achieve it. After that, execution is simply a matter of not giving up.

The objective is to get and stay functionally fit. So what's the key to functional fitness? Movement, or locomotion!

Locomotion: The Secret to Your Best Physique

Locomotion (or mobility) requires strength and ability. Locomotion is the skill of moving from one place to another. Synonyms include moving, traveling, mobility, progress, headway, action — you get the idea.

Locomotion is an important step in human growth during the transition from babies to toddlers. It's also one of the first we lose when we grow old. It's what you do every time you take a step, walk, run, sprint, climb, strike, throw, punch, kick, bowl, swing a club, get off the ground, or even get out of bed.

Locomotion is the ultimate function, because it is the single skill humans use most. It is the most necessary skill to our survival and well-being. More than anything else in existence, locomotion impacts our health and fitness.

Okay, so how do you improve this important skill that allows you to look and feel your best?

Understand locomotion

First you need to understand how humans absorb, transfer, and generate force to get from place to place, without wasted effort.

I spent two decades studying locomotion firsthand (with athletes and their trainers), observing it (particularly how different people move in different cultures), and applying it to survive (as a Special Operations trainer, a warrior, and as a pro fighter).

I didn't want to add to the sports science Tower of Babel. Instead, I sought to reduce locomotion down to its simplest nature, by formulating a fundamental strategy of how humans can move better.

Improve locomotion as quickly as possible

How do you improve this most vital skill as quickly as you can? By simplifying. And that's the secret to this program.

I first unveiled my strategy in Zurich, Switzerland, in 2018: The strongest and leanest bodies are best achieved through moving your hips and shoulders around a neutrally aligned spine, in a coordinated manner, which results in side-to-side weight shifting.

Okay, now I realize that doesn't sound very simple, does it? But don't worry, I've done the hard work to distill it all down into simple body movements that will improve your locomotion as fast as your body safely can.

Your Body Is a Tower

If someone built a tower out of balloons, you'd probably think twice before putting an office on the fifth floor. Building your best body is indeed like building a tower. Only by understanding and applying the fundamentals to athletic ability and strength can you build a structure capable of supporting yourself.

Your body's ability to resist stress depends on its alignment

Human bodies are essentially bunches of sticks (bones) stacked vertically. It's a marvel they stand up on their own!

Think of your body as a tall radio tower held up by cables extending to the ground. If all the cables are perfectly proportioned and taut, the tower stands straight and strong.

But if a single cable is unstable and not in tune with the others, the whole tower can topple. When this happens to your body, your brain sends out pain signals (in your knees, back, hips, neck, shoulders, etc.) and your posture starts going awry. The key is to develop a program that strengthens and integrates all these "cables."

Ideal joint alignment

The long-term integrity and strength needed to safely withstand day-to-day stress come from the ideal alignment of your parts. Posture and ideal joint alignment determine performance in all we do.

Making this look simple took me years. Unlike a tower or a building, which are static structures, your body's alignment is a fluid and constantly changing thing.

Spinal stabilization

Achieving your best body requires the ability to move your arms and legs around a neutral and stable spine. That's why most days you'll first use a floor exercise to stabilize your spine. You're then challenged to move your arms and legs around that stable spine. Lastly, after being prepared by the floor and mobility exercises, you can put it all together where it counts most, which is in the standing exercises.

Joint functions

When a joint is in the middle of its range of motion (neutrally aligned), it is in the safest position, since it's farthest away from the extreme ranges of motion. Here all movement options are more readily available, which increases your preparedness to safely move in all directions.

Most strength-training programs don't consider this, and you therefore lose a lot of joint functions. Heavy squatters, for example, often lose some internal hip rotation. Too much bench pressing can lead to forward head posture and rounded shoulders. When bodyweight exercises are not balanced properly, they can lead to injury.

Weight shifting

Improving balance is less about maintaining awkward static positions and much more about control of rhythmic side-to-side weight shifting. It's an important advantage to have, with vastly greater carryover to improved performance in real life. Humans rarely stand still in awkward positions. Instead, anytime we move, we use side-to-side weight shifting — walking, running, crawling, climbing, jumping, striking, throwing, getting groceries, lifting children, carrying things, you name it.

Focusing on Developmental Movements

These are the movements that you learned early in life, the ones that allowed you to move your entire body from one place to another.

Babies learn to stabilize their spines early on. They then learn to move their arms and legs (hip and shoulder functions) in random combinations until one of them resulted in a lateral weight shift that allowed them to transition from a back lying to a side lying position. For a baby, this triggers an instant and powerful reward, prompting more of the same behavior. This continues until the child can get into the front lying, crawling, and eventually standing positions.

It is in the transitions between lying, kneeling, sitting, and standing positions that the essential fundamental skills of human movement are learned. This is the athletic skill set acquired first in life, and when it begins to deteriorate later in life, our quality of life deteriorates proportionately. Maintaining the ability to transition between lying and standing positions with efficiency is the key to maintaining locomotion, and therefore fitness.

Mobility

It doesn't do you a lot of good to be super strong at a few exercise in the gym if you're too stiff to do common day-to-day activities, which is why I prioritize mobility — your ability to position properly — over muscle strength in one area. Your quality of life greatly depends on your mobility: The ability to get into the right position.

Stability

Stability is your ability to maintain positions, especially while force is acting against you, which is also a good description of strength. Developing an athletic and good looking body is about developing the mobility to position properly, and then developing the stability to maintain that ideal alignment in increasingly difficult situations, so you can remain safe and efficient.

Essentially, improving athleticism is about increasing your stress tolerance by improving your ability to safely absorb force.

Force absorption

"Use the force, Luke" —Obi-Wan Kenobi.

As we go through life there are constant forces acting against us, which we have to learn to handle skillfully. As a primary example, the force of gravity is applied to your body 24 hours a day.

While walking, sitting, swimming, and sleeping, your body is adapting to the forces acting against it. When you exercise, you are consciously applying force to your body in a specific way in order to bring about some kind of positive change. If done incorrectly, you'll eventually get hurt. If done in a balanced and systematic way, you will become more stress tolerant.

However, that increased stress tolerance isn't just the result of bigger and stronger muscles, it's also the result of learning how to move and position yourself in a way that allows force to be evenly distributed throughout your body.

Load sharing

Load sharing is the concept of evenly distributing the force of a load, so that stress is not unnecessarily concentrated in any particular area. Even distribution of force allows you to do more with less chance of injury. As an example, if you have a five-person team carrying a heavy log, that team will perform best when all members are working equally and in unison.

Likewise, the parts of your body are like the members of a team that must learn to work together and coordinate their efforts in order to make things as easy as possible. Force can be absorbed safely and efficiently by being distributed as evenly and broadly as possible through your body.

Perfect posture and physique

The athletes I've worked with have incredible physiques, not because they can throw heavy weights around, but because they're skilled at performing movements properly and efficiently. They perfectly balance stability and mobility, only moving the body parts that need to be moved while not moving the other parts.

Being good at other exercises will not ensure you can plow through the movements in this book. Performing them well requires the skill to build the best physique. They also help fitness newcomers improve strength and muscle tone quickly and safely, and they help those looking to lose weight shed those unwanted pounds. You'll be astonished how quickly you can progress into advanced levels.

Your Performance Pyramid

The height of your performance pyramid depends on the strength and breadth of your foundation. If you want to build a very tall and lasting structure, you need an extremely strong foundation. Likewise, the height of your performance will depend on the strength of your athletic fundamentals that make up your foundation. The best athletes always work on the basics. It might not sound sexy, but it is absolutely necessary.

TIP

Longevity and long-term success is all about the attention you give to the fundamentals. Your ability to maintain good posture, move your arms and legs around a neutral spine, control weight shifting, and get and up down from the ground all determine your athleticism, now and forever.

Avoid neglect

The great thing about getting so specific about your most basic and essential needs is that it allows you to do what's necessary with a minimum of wasted energy. Simply by doing the floor exercises in this book, you will improve and maintain your posture and joint functions, which are the foundation of everything. Neglect is unlikely when the payoff is so high and the sacrifice so small.

Aging does not equal disabling

Aging is a normal and unavoidable part of life. However, disability and unnecessary suffering can be avoidable. By drilling and refining the movements you learned first in life, you can improve your movement and mobility, even very late in life.

Living Pain Free

Pain can come from over-exercising, or exercising the wrong way, just as it can come from not exercising at all. Developing a program that seeks to create your leanest and strongest body, while keeping you pain free, and even helping eradicate current pain, is a science.

Coordination helps you avoid injury

Because they take coordination in the real world out of the equation, fitness machines often make you good at using fitness machines and not much else.

In fact, there have been times I've mistakenly thought some of my clients were disabled until I learned they were trainers who exclusively used fitness machines. Machines limit your movement options and can therefore impair your coordination. Contraptions don't train your body to function as a cohesive whole outside of the gym, and so you are more likely to develop ineffective motor patterns. Too often that can lead to injury.

Functional exercises are the safest

Just as it's no coincidence that the most functional exercises produce the most desirable bodies, it's also no coincidence that the most functional exercises are almost always the safest. They keep the tower of your body perfectly aligned, so nothing is sending out alarm calls of pain before toppling.

Because of this, in a matter of weeks, many of my clients have eradicated knee, hip, shoulder, and neck pain.

Lessen hip and knee pain

Knees were made to kneel. So why, then, does simply kneeling on a hard surface hurt so many people? Because unlike our ancestors, many people have grown very unused to kneeling. Remember the old adage, "use it or lose it"?

But when you kneel properly, you engage your leg and core muscles to control the motion, to bring your kneecap down gently. This builds and strengthens not just your leg muscles, but your core muscles as well.

It's fine to exercise with a yoga mat. But I'm finding more and more of my clients don't need them. I personally use the polished concrete floor in my condo. This forces my body to kneel down properly. It's one of the secrets to eradicating knee pain.

TIP

During these exercises, keep your feet parallel to one another. Make sure your toes do not point out. Imagine a line going from the center of your heel to the center of *all five toes* (not your big toe!). Place your feet so these lines run parallel. This may feel strange at first, but it's vital for proper knee alignment. Keep your knees pointing in the same direction as your toes.

Systematically training all the different functions of your hips — a focal point of this program — is essential to having healthy and flexible hips.

Ameliorate lower back, neck, and shoulder pain

It's amazing how many of your common aches and pains can be resolved within weeks, simply by training all the functions of your joints. The movements that make up the floor exercises in Chapter 4 cover the movements of your hips, spine, and shoulders. If you're suffering from pain, doing just 4-8 reps of each exercise once a week is often enough to correct the muscular imbalances that cause that pain. Then you can progress to doing two sets per exercise and eventually move pain free through the mobility exercises in Chapter 10.

Putting the Building Blocks of Calisthenics in Place

This section defines some basic terms that you need to know in order to start an exercise program.

- » **Reps:** Single repetitions. If you do ten push-ups, that's ten reps.
- » **Sets:** If you do ten push-ups, then rest, that's one set of push-ups. Sets can be made up of any number of reps, but typically range from 5-15.
- » **Rests:** Breaks in between sets.
- » **Workouts:** What you do in a single session on any given day.
- » **Cycles:** After a few weeks of workouts, you'll complete a cycle. And then you can move on to the next one!

TIP

Reps (like letters) are combined into *sets* (like words), with *rests* between (like spaces). This then forms *workouts* (like sentences). *Cycles* are paragraphs. And together, these form the book of your body, your life.

>> **Rest and recovery:** Your muscles don't strengthen while you are working out. They strengthen while you rest. The more muscle you build, the more fat you burn — but always when you're at rest.

While light, steady-state activities such as walking, jogging, or light calisthenics are not ideal for making you leaner, they are useful for improving movement quality and recovery. Some light activity on your rest days is a great way to speed up recovery. With that said, first and foremost is sleep and relaxation.

Take time to chill out and avoid doing too many unnecessary things. It's true what they say in Thai boxing: "Champions are lazy."

Focusing on Attention and Breathing

By now you've obviously noticed my obsession with the fundamentals, which are the things constantly in use. I've mentioned posture, joint functions, and weight shifting. However, there are skills even more basic than these. And so for that reason they're even more important. Your attention and breath are the basics that are always in use, without exception. And just like your limbs, you can learn to control them.

REMEMBER

Buddha primarily taught two things: to focus on their breath, and to move their attention through their different body parts. Like meditation, fitness is all about focus.

Listen to your limbs. Feel where they are in space and in relation to each other. Feel how they respond to the stress you apply. The more intuitively you can do this, the more you will perfect your form, and the fitter you will become.

Syncing your breathing with your movements is also vital. Inhale on the negative half of the movement (for example, as your chest descends to the floor in a push-up). Exhale on the positive portion of the movement (as you push yourself off the ground). Your breathing sets the pace for your reps.

Performance Leads to Efficiency

Another advantage of not working out in a gym: No one's watching you. No pressure to lift more or faster than you should.

When I sent trainers my exercises ahead of my earliest certification courses, some told me they found them easy. I thought, "Yikes, I must be getting old!" I find these tough. Then I'd show up and they'd proudly crank out reps for me, but with poor posture. When I corrected them, it drastically changed the difficulty of the movements, as well as the benefits they reaped. As I've seen again and again, even the seemingly simplest exercise is difficult if you do it with the right form.

You only get good at what you do

It was my boxing training in Thailand that drove this lesson home. I would see teenage Thai boxers manhandle much bigger and "stronger" men. These Thai boxers could stand directly in front of me and land a shin on my neck. Yet when it came to static stretching — which only the foreigners did — they could barely touch their own toes! It blew my mind.

I realized I wouldn't get good at Thai boxing by doing curls and hitting the Stairmaster. Instead, I became a professional Thai boxing champion by practicing Thai boxing. It seems obvious, right? But our society too often wrongly equates strength in the gym with performance in real life and real sports.

The most effective way to train for something is simply by doing the actual thing you're training for.

Focus on the fundamentals

As any jujitsu master will tell you, learn just a few fundamental holds perfectly, and no one will ever be able to defeat you. This is a primary reason people spend far too long working out, yet do not getting the results they want. They're not training with proper form, and so they are not perfecting the fundamentals.

REMEMBER

Focusing on the fundamentals of locomotion and training them with proper form is the quickest route to achieving your best body.

Mastery of life

How do you become good at not just Thai boxing or bench pressing or running, but the ability to move through life like an athlete?

As a young Special Ops guy, it was my job to be ready for all types of missions and environments at a moment's notice. On any given training cycle, we might jump out of the back of a plane at 12,000 feet, wearing 130 pounds of gear and night vision goggles, skydiving after Harley-Davidson dirt bikes they'd just chucked out — strapped to pallets with parachutes attached — which we'd use the instant we hit the ground to practice rapid airfield seizures. A day later, we could be diving off the shores of Hawaii. And then summiting Mount Rainier the same week. We had to be ready for everything.

I noticed that as I focused on one skill, the others would quickly weaken. If I ran a lot, my strength would decrease. If I focused on strength training, my running and swimming would suffer.

My first obvious lesson came immediately after graduating from the Pararescue/Combat Control Indoctrination Course, one of the toughest selection courses in the military. I strapped on a 60-pound pack for the first time. The week before, I had broken the military's underwater record by swimming 133 meters subsurface in a single breath. By almost any measure, I was in superhuman condition, but I had never *rucked*, the military term for walking with a heavy pack.

The lesson was instant and powerful. I could barely keep up with my peers, whom I had easily outpaced in every other event during selection. All that training was for nothing when it came to getting from point A to point B with gear.

This environment ingrained in me a constant need to simplify and reduce, so that problems can be solved with minimal effort by focusing only on the essentials. And when I took command of the physical training on my base, I worked hard to make training smarter and less complicated. These lessons allowed me to cut through the complexity and nonsense of the fitness industry as well.

If you only get good at what you do, how is it possible to create an exercise program that effectively prepares you for just about everything? For life itself? This is the functional training riddle that has gone unanswered for too long.

The answer: by isolating and focusing on the precise, specific fundamentals needed for locomotion. This means, with only 20-30 minutes a day, you can indeed get better at everything. You'll be amazed at how little you need to do to achieve your best body, your best *you*.

Chapter **3**

Setting Goals and Staying Motivated

We asked 1,000 people, men and women from all 50 states, "What motivates you to work out?" We learned what works and what doesn't. But a few people actually stated that they simply would *not* work out unless someone gave them "cold hard cash"! Although bodyweight training often increases energy and focus, this is unfortunately a book, and not an ATM. So, instead, here are real-world, tried-and-true methods proven to keep you on track and achieve your best body.

Knowing What You Want from a Calisthenics Program

You picked up this book with a goal in mind. Perhaps you want to lose weight. Maybe you want to build muscle and get stronger. Maybe you want to start a fitness routine, but aren't ready or willing to head to a gym. Those are all acceptable reasons to start a calisthenics program.

To achieve success with a bodyweight training program, it's best to know what you want out of it. The following sections help you clarify your goals and stay motivated.

Evaluate where you are and where you want to be

You already have this book in your hands — a simple tool to get you into the best shape of your life. That is a very real, attainable goal. Consistently training and eating properly will get you there. It really is that simple. The only thing that can stop you from getting there is you.

But you probably won't get there if you don't know where "there" is. So what exactly are your goals?

Maybe you want to be able to lift your luggage without a problem. Or lift your grandchildren. Or run a mile without getting winded. Or even just walk one. Think of one to three goals like this that you want to achieve.

TIP

Your ability to achieve and maintain higher levels of fitness is dependent on the amount of attention and value you give to the *essentials*:

>> Breathing and posture

>> Tensing and relaxing your muscles

>> Focusing on your joint positions and muscle actions in developmental movements

>> Training and recovery

>> And most of all, doing all those things consistently

Although it's less quantifiable, your main goal should be to improve your awareness and understanding of these skills. Try to notice how improving these basics improves everything else in your life. After all, fundamentals are fundamentals because they are the things most often in use. You'll be shocked by the benefit in terms of how you look, feel, and move. Bring your attention to the most common and basic movements. That's what real fitness is all about.

Create specific goals

You need to make your goals specific, measurable, and quantifiable. That way, each goal gives you a bull's-eye to aim for.

TIP

Your goals should answer at least these questions:

>> How much of something do you want to gain, lose, or do?

>> What is your timeline?

Many people start with goals that are too general. An example of a general goal is "I want to be fitter." On the surface, that's an admirable goal. But how will you know when you're more fit? And how fit do you want to get? If this is your goal, you can't easily answer those questions. That's why you need to be more specific. Consider these examples:

>> Start my first workout this Monday.

>> For one week, cut sugary drinks from my diet and replace them with water.

>> Perform all the floor exercises with proper form by my birthday.

>> Go one whole program without missing a workout.

These goals are specific. They have a measurable outcome to reach by a certain date.

TIP

Take the goal or goals you came up with in the preceding section and make them more specific. Add a timeline and a measurement of achievement. Now write them down! Having them in writing, to look at whenever you need, is a great step to not only making them real, but achieving them.

Step away from the scale

Losing 5, 10, 20, 40, or even more pounds of fat is an admirable, realistic goal. But remember, it's all about body composition, not simply pounds. Muscle weighs more than fat. If you lose fat but gain muscle, the scales only shows the balance between the two, not the pounds of fat you lost. That's why a scale can be an incredibly poor indicator of progress.

If you follow this program, you *will* attain realistic goals, and the best, realistic figure for your own personal body. How long it takes to get there depends on how far away you are. Consider the following real-world examples:

>> Sarah was a pretty fit, 140-pound female at 25 percent body fat. After two months on our program, she replaced six pounds of fat with three pounds of muscle. So while she lost six pounds of fat, the scale told her she lost only three pounds total body weight, which is true. In two months, she changed her body-fat percentage from 25 to 20 percent. This overall change in body weight of only three pounds

gave her a significant reduction in body fat! All while *increasing* her metabolism with new muscle.

Sarah's change in body composition was relatively easy yet significant. It improved her appearance, metabolism, athleticism, and her overall ability to make continued progress.

>> John weighed in at 230. He began our strength training program, stuck to it for two months, stepped on the scale every day, and then became discouraged that he had only lost nine pounds after 60 days of training. He weighed 221 pounds, hardly where he wanted to be. He could hardly see the three pounds of muscle he gained because he still had a lot of fat masking them. His morale took a nose dive, and before you know it, he succumbed to any excuse not to workout. He gained the weight back and continued his long, slow descent into obesity.

John's actually made better progress than the thinner Sarah, although it wasn't apparent to the naked eye. What John did not realize is that, while he lost fat, he also gained strength. It may not sound like much, but he made a significant change in his body composition. He lost 12 pounds of fat and added 3 pounds of muscle. This increased his metabolism, setting him up for continued success. If John continued to work out, this success would only snowballs as he accrued more muscle, could train more intensely, and then would burn more fat per week as time went on. For John, who has a lot of weight to lose, it will take time. But it *will* happen.

The weight increase from muscle gained will slow after these first three months of strength training, while the weight decrease from fat lost will also increase, but more slowly as well.

This is quite different from what most people do. Usually people lose fat while also losing more muscle than necessary. That may satisfy the need to see a smaller number on the scale, but it doesn't lead to a strong, healthy physique.

You can and will have the kind of body you want, but if you're far from your goal, for the change to be real and lasting, you must be patient. Slow and steady wins the race.

I know: *It sucks.* Waiting sucks. But it's simply impossible to magically undo ten years of neglect in two months. Nothing can do that for you. No pills, contraptions, or diets. With this program, you'll lose fat and build muscle to make sure it doesn't come back.

A pound of muscle takes up about half the space of a pound of fat. So if you lose three pounds of fat around your waist, that decrease will show much more than the slight increase in your muscles, which leads to firmer triceps and legs.

See your effort pay off

TIP

A better indicator of your progress than a scale is how your clothes fit. Over time, you'll start to see changes. Your clothes will fit you better. And whether they tell you or not, people around you will notice. As you continue to train, you'll see the results: New lines, a new shape, the curves of growing muscles, a hardness you didn't have before. Your body will change. With consistency, you'll start to look better.

For almost everyone I know, *results* are the ultimate motivator. When you start to see a change in your physique, your effort and positive attitude gain momentum. Seeing is believing.

Embrace the mental boost

Pay attention to your mood and attitude too. Embrace the times when you feel great after working out, when it seems to calm your mind and reduce stress, and when you feel a boost just because you are caring for yourself. You are choosing to be good to yourself and that feels good. Remember how this feels. It can get you through the tough times.

Throwing Your Ego Out with the Weights

It's not just your body weight, but weights themselves that are not a sole measure of success. If you're not in the gym, there's no one to try to impress by grabbing a bigger weight plate.

However, even when they make the switch to bodyweight movements, so many people only want to do the hardest possible exercises. Yet they lack the fundamentals to execute them properly.

Let me tell you the secret to your best body, one that differentiates elite athletes from those who wish they were:

Form = Physique

Worry less about how much weight or how many reps you can do and focus instead on keeping proper form while doing those reps. Performing exercises while maintaining ideal joint alignment ensures that you're training the intended muscles while improving coordination, balance, posture, and joint functions — which are the things that make you look and feel your best. This is the route to achieving a beautiful, strong body that can last into old age.

The true measure of your merit

The plan is to make you stronger, leaner, and more mobile while teaching you to move properly in order to increase your performance and injury resistance in real life. It's all about movement quality, which is your ability to position yourself properly so you can maintain ideal joint alignment when you're not exercising.

REMEMBER

For all exercises, the challenge is to make yourself as long and straight as possible, through all parts of your body, while using a full range of motion, breathing rhythmically, and staying relaxed.

The true measure of merit is your ability to make it look good! Humans naturally have an eye and desire for athletic ability, which is recognizable when a person moves with long straight lines, with a steady cadence and a sense of effortlessness.

Start small and progress gradually

The best advice for starting a calisthenics program is to take it one step at a time.

If you're unfamiliar with a certain type of training or it's been a while since you've worked out, it takes very little effort to make progress. Many people don't believe how little is needed, especially when you're doing the right things, which is why the most common fitness mistake is doing too much, especially in the beginning.

WARNING

Don't start off by doing too much. You risk injury, might end up being so sore that it's demotivating, and you might just hate every minute of it. Keep it light and stay consistent. A light, ten-minute workout on your living room floor is enough to get started. It can feel hard, but if it hurts, stop doing it. You should experience a little muscle soreness. About 24–48 hours later you'll be fully recovered, a little bit stronger, and ready to do it again.

With calisthenics, small steps reap big rewards.

Finding and Keeping Your Motivation

Motivation is a big factor in whether you stick to your workout and meet your fitness goals. When starting a fitness program, you may need to force yourself to exercise. After you establish a routine and start seeing results, you'll be more motivated to continue. Then it becomes cyclical: Success leads to more motivation, which leads to more success, which leads to more motivation. You get the idea. The following sections explain how this works.

Every Monday morning (or whenever your "workout week" begins), tell yourself, *out loud*, that you will do your workouts that week. Be specific. Tell yourself that you will work out on your chosen three days. For example, "I will complete this week's workouts on Monday, Wednesday, and Friday." It sounds funny, but a simple declaration like this can increase physical activity.

Big rewards, small costs

Subconsciously, people are always weighing the *rewards versus costs* to decide whether or not to repeat any activity.

This is one of the great benefits of calisthenics: In the time it takes you to get to the gym, you can already be done with your workout. That's huge! You can get much more out of it in the same time and that makes the behavior addictive. Start small and increase gradually. Successful training of any type is more about playful and consistent repetition than anything else. Enjoy yourself.

As you progress in your workouts, your movement will become stronger, and your real-life performance will increase significantly, which will further motivate you to stay consistent. Lasting motivation is about rewards and improved efficiency so you can get more for less.

A short workout can pay enormous dividends: Your stress is washed away, your mind and body are revitalized, your self-esteem is lifted, and those feel-good endorphins explode through your body. This pays off in spades.

Independence day

So much of what people have learned about fitness only hinders their potential. Unrealistic expectations, "no pain, no gain," pushing to injury, and more. Don't let fear of dumbbells, machines, or gadgets prevent you from reaching your optimum level of fitness. You don't need them!

You can certainly do this program with a buddy, and having someone to motivate you can make the program more fun and less daunting. The only danger is that your workout partner might back out some day. Will you be able to carry on without them? You don't want that to become your excuse not to work out. Most of the truly fit men and women I know are the ones who do it by themselves.

Only *you* know what you need and when you need it. Only *you* feel your muscles, lungs, bones, and ligaments. In the end, only *you* can get you into shape. And that's all you need: You.

Making your health a top priority

As mentioned, making your health a priority is a kindness you give yourself. It takes effort, but you are worth it. By buying this book, you have begun the journey. When you are fit, you can meet life's obstacles with physical and mental strength.

TIP

If you want detailed video tutorials for many of the exercises in this book, go to the Instagram page *Mark_Lauren_Bodyweight*. You'll find a link in the bio that gives you access to all the free videos in the subscription app, called Mark Lauren On Demand.

Overcoming Obstacles

Up to this point in the chapter, we've given you some tools for a successful journey to your best body. You also need to be ready for obstacles so you can effectively combat them, which is what this section covers.

Dealing with injuries

WARNING

Consult your doctor before you begin an exercise regimen, especially if you suffer from any kind of injury.

Many common ailments can be corrected and prevented by systematically training your joint functions with relatively easy exercises.

TIP

If you're suffering from pain, start with exercises that you can perform easily, and then increase the difficulty gradually. This is what the floor exercises covered in Chapter 4 are for. If you find that those exercises are too difficult, download the Mark Lauren Bodyweight Training app and use the Prep Program, which will build you from the ground up with rehabilitation type movements.

Modifying your routine when life gets in the way

It doesn't take much to maintain a basic fitness level. On the occasion when an emergency vanquishes your free time, two to three short sessions a week is enough to keep you healthy and resilient.

When stress increases because of travel, increased workloads, illness, or other factors, don't compound your problems by exercising harder than you have to. Exercise is a form of stress as well, and it can injure you or make you sick, especially when environmental factors are turning up the heat.

Picking up where you left off

You may experience some false starts as you begin your journey as a strong, fit person. The important thing is to try, try again. Change is hard and we don't always succeed the first time. What's important is to get back at it. Be kind to yourself, leave the guilt behind, and restart your routine. Your behavior *now* directly affects your behavior in the future. Make winning a habit.

Your commitment and resolve will improve as you stick with it and begin to see results.

Facing Down Your Excuses

When something is hard (and change is hard), it's easy to come up with excuses not to do it. That's human. I have to work late, so I can't work out. I don't have enough energy to work out. My dog hid my sneakers (okay, you'd probably realize that excuse when you utter it).

Ultimately, you have to decide that your physical and mental health are more important.

Giving in to your excuses backfires

Being even moderately fit by adding 20-30 minutes of exercise to your life four times a week can lighten your mood, lessen anxiety, fight off depression, help with insomnia, heal back pain, address low bone density, increase mobility, lower heart disease, and combat obesity.

Those are significant benefits for only 1 percent of your week! If you let your excuses take over, you can't reap the benefits of any of this.

TIP

Try writing down the daily excuses that prevent you from reaching your goals. Do it in two columns — goals and excuses side by side — so you can see how often you obstruct your goals with your excuses.

Common excuses we hear include:

>> I don't have time.

>> I'm too tired.

>> I'm in a bad mood.

>> I don't feel like it.

>> I need to relax.

>> It's too hard.

>> I'll start over next week.

>> I'll make up for it.

After you've written your excuses down, take a look at them. Decide now that when you hear these thoughts again, you're going to work out despite them.

Resisting your excuses creates a better you

As mentioned, there are hundreds of benefits to regularly following an effective physical training program, but one that is often overlooked is your improved ability to serve others. Your friends, loved ones, and coworkers will get a stronger version of you. Take the time to serve yourself, so you can better serve others. That, above all, is beautiful.

While there is no actual fountain of youth, exercise has been proven over and over again to be the best thing for maintaining health, fitness, and a youthful attitude. Becoming a stronger, leaner you now paves the way for a brighter, stronger future for all those around you. If you care about their happiness, first care about your own.

This is your time

It helps most people to set a specific time to exercise each day. Find a time — morning, lunch break, evening — and stick to it.

WARNING

Don't think, "I'll wait and see if I have time," or "I'll try to squeeze it in later." Most likely, it just won't happen. Make a date with yourself. Then hold yourself accountable. The great thing about calisthenics is that it can happen whenever is best for your schedule.

There will never be the "perfect" time or condition to work out. You have to create the time because you decide you are worth it.

TIP

Turn your phone off. Forget about work, family, friends, and anything that can get in your way of achieving a better, healthier life. Don't worry, when you're done, you'll return to the world more energized and stronger than ever, ready to tackle just about anything. The world can wait. Right here, right now, this is *your time*.

2

The Exercises

Chapter **4**

Getting Down with Floor Exercises

I n this chapter, you learn all about floor exercises, including the specific benefits of the different exercises. The chapter starts by laying out the advantages you'll gain from back lying, crawling, front lying, and side lying exercises. Then it gets into the practical part — the actual exercises!

WARNING It's always a good idea to check with your doctor before you begin an exercise regimen. Also, if any of the exercises in this chapter cause you pain, stop doing them. It's important to be able to recognize the difference between something that is hard and something that is painful. No exercise should cause pain. Always listen to your body.

Gaining Big Improvements with Small Exercises

The foundation of athletic ability and overall well-being depends largely on the health of your joints. Strength, flexibility, coordination, endurance, balance, and all other athletic qualities can only be developed to the degree that your joints are able to function properly, relatively pain free. In other words, no one is stronger than their joints. Fortunately, improving joint-health is simple and rewarding. Systematically training all the functions of your hips, spine, and shoulders is the foundation for a lifetime of pain-free training and long-term progress.

Developing better posture

Posture refers mainly to the alignment of your spine. "Good" posture is the position of your spine that allows for safe and effective absorption of force, which is typically long and relatively straight. When your spine is long and "straight," your vertebrae are stacked directly on top of one another and neutrally aligned, which leaves a margin of safety for movement in all directions. The opposite of being neutrally aligned, meaning aligned in the middle, is to be bent in any one direction. Obviously, if you are bent all the way forward, for example, your chances of injury are higher, because you are already at an extreme range of motion, with little room for error.

In order to improve posture, you need to learn to move your arms and legs around a properly aligned spine, which is easiest on the ground, in lying and crawling positions, where you have many points of contact with the ground. Simply put, there is less improvement of basic joint functions.

Improving hip, spine, and shoulder functions

These floor exercises were created with a checklist of joint functions to cover the hips, spine, and shoulders. We match up each of the items on our checklist with the best possible exercise to improve each function.

Better coordination means getting more for less

More than anything else, improved performance and stress tolerance depend on learning to do the right things while avoiding unnecessary movements. Your ability to master complex movements and activities depends largely on being able to isolate basic functions, so you can more easily recombine them in new ways. One of the important skills that floor exercises teach you is to move your body parts independent of one another.

Wondering how to incorporate all the exercises in this chapter into your week? Although your specific regimen might depend on your needs and any injuries you're nursing, you can start by using this simple schedule to incorporate these floor exercises into your week:

Monday: Back lying exercises

Tuesday: Side lying exercises

Thursday: Front lying exercises

Friday: Crawling exercises

Start by doing 4-8 reps of each exercise. Once that becomes too easy, do two sets of 4-8 reps of each movement.

Back Lying Exercises

The back lying exercises focus mainly on core and hip strength while improving your posture. You can make these exercises harder by keeping your legs straight.

Dead bugs

This exercise helps you feel long and straight while teaching you to control front to back pelvic tilting, which is what controls the arch in your lower back. If you want to prevent and/or reduce lower back pain, this is an essential skill. The key to doing this exercise correctly is to keep your lower back in contact with the ground throughout the movement.

1. **Lie down on your back with your arms above your shoulders and your knees above your hips.**

   Your hips, knees, and ankles should be bent at 90 degree angles, as shown in Figure 4-1a. It's important to keep the knees directly over the hips, so that you're challenged to use your abdominals instead of a mechanical advantage. Tighten your midsection and draw your navel in toward your spine to keep your lower back on the ground.

2. **From this starting position, fully extend the left leg with your knees and toes pointing straight up, as shown in Figure 4-1b.**

   Make yourself as long and straight as possible while keeping the other parts of your body perfectly still. Extending your leg makes it more difficult to keep your lower back pressed into the ground, which is why it improves control of front to back pelvic tilting.

3. **Reset to the starting position to complete one rep on the left side.**

   Get into a perfect starting position as described in Step 1 before beginning the next rep.

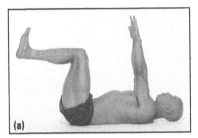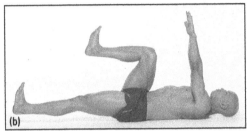

Photo by Jorge Alvarez, www.alvarezphoto.com

FIGURE 4-1:
The dead bugs exercise, starting position (a) and final position (b).

TIP

As you do this exercise, imagine a training partner trying to slide their hand under your back. If you're doing the movement correctly, your lower back should be firmly pressed into ground preventing them from doing so!

Glute hip-ups

Almost everything you do in life involves stepping, which requires simultaneous hip flexion and extension. Improving the strength and flexibility for these movements has a big payoff for that reason. This exercise strengthens your glutes (your rear end) while stretching your hip flexors (top front of your thighs).

1. **Lie down on your back with your arms at your sides, palms up.**

   Pull your left foot to your hips and pull your right knee to your chest, as in Figure 4-2a.

2. **While keeping your right knee actively pulled in toward your chest, raise your hips as high as possible by squeezing the left glute and driving the left foot into the ground, as in Figure 4-2b.**

3. **Lower yourself fully to complete one rep on the left side.**

FIGURE 4-2:
Starting position
for glute hip-ups
(a) and final
position (b),
where you raise
your hips as high
as possible while
actively pulling
your knee into
your chest.

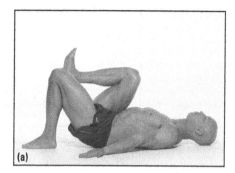
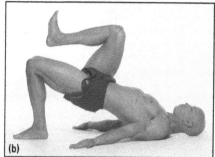

Photo by Jorge Alvarez, www.alvarezphoto.com

TIP

Keeping the elevated knee actively pulled into your chest prevents you from arching through your lower back, which protects your lower spine and strengthens your posture.

Up and overs

This a great full body exercise that emphasizes core strength and improved joint alignment. One of the key elements of this movement is challenging you to control hip rotation while making yourself as long and straight as possible.

1. **Lie down on your back with your arms at the T position and your legs fully extended, as shown in Figure 4-3a.**

    Keep your toes and knees pointing straight up throughout this exercise — that means control hip rotation!

2. **Pull your left knee in toward your chest while reaching up to the sky with your left arm, as shown in Figure 4-3b.**

3. **Lower your left leg and left arm back to the starting position, as shown in Figure 4-3c.**

4. **Then reach across your body to the right with your left hand while pulling your left knee to your chest, as shown in Figure 4-3d.**

5. **Reset to the starting position to complete the rep.**

Making yourself long and straight as you pull a knee to your chest requires that you fully extend the opposite leg, which tends to cause external hip rotation. It is your mission to keep the knee of the extended leg pressed into the ground with the knee cap pointing straight up. Better control of hip rotation will improve your joint alignment for basic activities like walking and running.

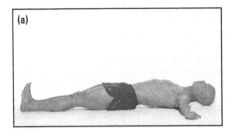
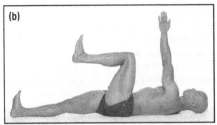
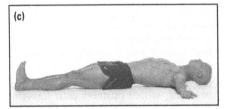
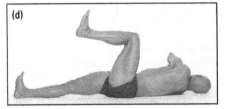

FIGURE 4-3:
The up and
over is a great
full-body
exercise.

Photo by Jorge Alvarez, www.alvarezphoto.com

Windshield wipers

This exercise strengthens your hips and core while improving spinal rotation.

1. **Lie down on your back with your arms at the T position and your knees directly above your hips.**

   Keep your hips, knees, and ankles bent at 90 degree angles throughout the exercise, as shown in Figure 4-4a.

2. **Lower your left leg to the left side until it almost touches the ground, as shown in Figure 4-4b. Then lower the right leg to the left leg.**

3. **Lastly, reverse the movement by raising the right leg, and then raise the left leg back to the original starting position.**

   If you're doing this exercise correctly, only one leg should be moving at any one time.

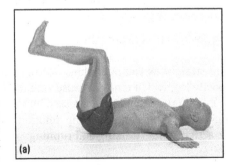
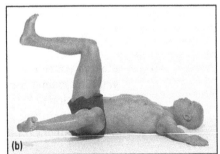

FIGURE 4-4:
The windshield
wipers exercise
involves moving
one leg at a time.

Photo by Jorge Alvarez, www.alvarezphoto.com

As you do this exercise, work on keeping both shoulders on the ground. This will challenge your flexibility so you can learn to move your hips independently of your shoulders and rotate more freely around your spine.

Crawling Exercises

Crawling exercises focus mainly on your glutes by improving hip functions. Focus on getting a full range of motion with every rep. You can increase the difficulty of these exercises by increasing the size of your movements.

Dirty dogs

Dirty dogs improve external hip rotation and work the upper part of your glutes, which allow you to rotate your leg outward.

1. **Get into a crawling position with your hands on the ground directly beneath your shoulders, arms straight, and left knee slightly elevated.**

   Your ankles, knees, and hips should be at about 90 degree angles, as shown in Figure 4-5a.

2. **Raise the left knee straight out to the side and as high as possible while maintaining the same bend in your knee and ankle, as shown in Figure 4-5b.**

   Only your left leg should be moving. The rest of your body should be still while maintaining a crawling position.

TIP

For crawling movements, make yourself stable and comfortable by positioning yourself so that your shoulders are directly over your wrists and your hips are pushed slightly back behind your knees. Most people find that this position is easiest on the wrists and knees while providing good stability.

FIGURE 4-5:
Starting position (a) and ending position (b) for dirty dogs.

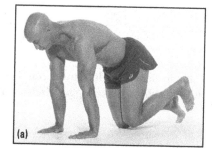
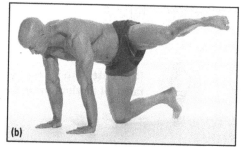

Photo by Jorge Alvarez, www.alvarezphoto.com

Hip circles

This movement teaches you to make big circles with your hips, which allow you to move your legs in a circular motion. Hip circles are great for overall hip mobility and the development of your upper glutes.

1. Start from a crawling position with your left knee slightly elevated off the ground, as shown in Figure 4-6a.

2. Raise the left knee toward your left elbow, as shown in Figure 4-6b.

3. Continue to raise the left knee as high as possible in a circular motion going backward, as shown in Figure 4-6c.

4. Lower the left knee while continuing to move in a circular motion and reset to the starting position, as shown in Figure 4-6d.

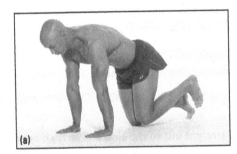
(a)

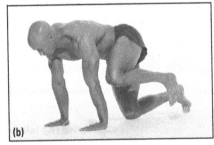
(b)

FIGURE 4-6: Hip circles are great for overall hip mobility and the development of your upper glutes.

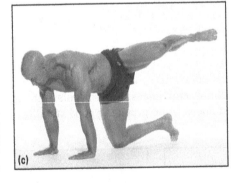
(c)

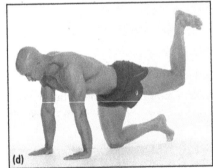
(d)

Photo by Jorge Alvarez, www.alvarezphoto.com

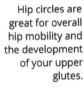

TIP

If you use both sides of your hips to raise your left knee, you'll get a much wider range of motion, meaning you'll be able to make bigger circles with your knee.

Pointers

The main function of pointers is to improve spinal flexion and extension (front-to-back bending). The exercise is a great standalone exercise to break up long periods of sitting, and it is especially useful as a preparation for standing leg movements, such as squats and lunges.

1. **Get into a crawling position. Make sure your hips are pushed back slightly behind your knees and that your shoulders are directly over your wrists, so that you're stable, as shown in Figure 4-7a.**

2. **Stabilize yourself with the right arms and left leg. Then bring your left elbow to your right knee while looking down at the ground, as shown in Figure 4-7b.**

3. **Straighten the left leg and right arm while also arching through your back and gently looking up. See Figure 4-7c.**

   Reset to the starting position to complete the rep.

Avoid swinging your limbs as you do this movement. You should be raising the opposite arm and leg in a controlled manner.

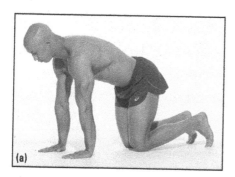
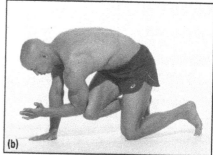
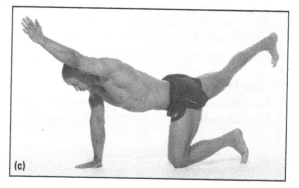

FIGURE 4-7: The pointers exercise improves spinal flexion and extension (front-to-back bending).

Photo by Jorge Alvarez, www.alvarezphoto.com

Straight wide legs

This is an excellent movement for your glutes that teaches you to control hip rotation. Most people tend to rotate their legs to the outside during hip extension and hip abduction.

With this exercise, you are being challenged to prevent external hip rotation while abducting a hip in an extended position. Developing this skill will allow you to maintain better joint alignment while taking big steps going forward and to the sides.

1. **Get into a crawling position with your left leg fully extended to the rear. Keep your left ankle flexed with your toes and knee pointing straight down at the ground, as shown in Figure 4-8a.**

2. **While keeping all other parts of your body perfectly still, move the elevated leg about six inches to the left, as shown in Figure 4-8b.**

Reset to the starting position to complete the repetition.

FIGURE 4-8:
Starting position (a) and ending position (b) of the straight wide leg exercise.

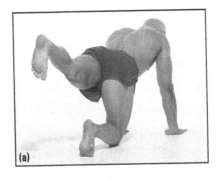 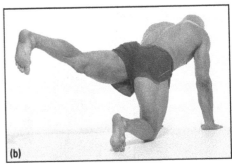

Photo by Jorge Alvarez, www.alvarezphoto.com

This is a short movement when done correctly. If you have a long range of motion, it is most likely because you are externally rotating the elevated leg and/or bending through your back. The toes and knee of the elevated leg should remain pointing straight down throughout the movement.

Straight wide legs are a great example of improving coordination by isolating functions. In this case, you are learning to move your legs away from center line, in an extended position, without hip rotation.

Front Lying Exercises

The main focus of the front lying exercises is to improve your shoulder and spine functions. To get the best possible benefit from these exercises, make yourself as long and straight possible, head to heels, while challenging yourself to get a full range of motion with each rep.

Hip twists

Hip twists build core strength while improving rotation of your lower spine.

1. **Get into a long straight push-up position, often called a *plank*.**

    Your shoulders should be directly above your wrists, and your feet need to be hip width apart, so that you can roll your hips in the next step without your feet stacking on top of each other, as shown in Figure 4-9a.

2. **While maintaining a straight line from head to heels, roll your heels all the way to the right, as shown in Figure 4-9b.**

    Both heels should touch the ground.

3. **Then roll your heels all the way to the left, as shown in Figure 4-9c.**

This is a nice movement for improving an often overlooked function of your spine and developing the front and sides of your midsection.

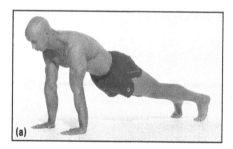
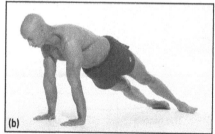
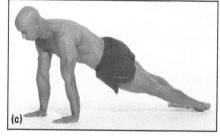

FIGURE 4-9: Hip twists help develop the front and sides of your midsection.

Photo by Jorge Alvarez, www.alvarezphoto.com

TIP

If you experience wrist pain from planking-type exercises or push-ups, try doing them on a hard surface without a mat. Using a mat, especially one that is thick and soft, increases the bend in your wrists, which can cause discomfort for that reason. You can also try turning your hands outward slightly so that your fingers are pointing away from your center line at about 45 degrees. This also decreases the bend in your wrists.

Moose antlers

Moose antlers are a great shoulder and thoracic spine mobility exercise that improve posture by getting your head into a better position.

1. **Lie down on your stomach with your right arm fully extended past your head and your left thumb on the back of your head, as shown in Figure 4-10a.**

2. **Crawl your right hand forward as far as you can, and then press it into the ground while raising the left elbow as high as possible, as shown in Figure 4-10b.**

   Make yourself as long as possible and exhale forcefully as you raise your elbow.

The main joint functions being trained with this exercise are shoulder extension and scapular retraction, which is especially good for activities like swimming, throwing, and turning your head while driving.

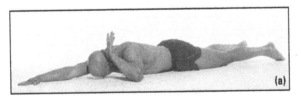

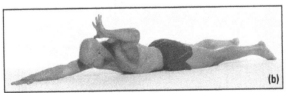

FIGURE 4-10: The moose antlers exercise helps your shoulder muscles.

Photo by Jorge Alvarez, www.alvarezphoto.com

Twists and reaches

The main function of this exercise is to improve rotation of the thoracic spine and shoulder mobility.

This excellent exercise is mainly intended to improve rotation of the thoracic spine, which is the part of your spine between mid-chest and the bottom of your neck. Like most of these floor exercises, the twist and reach is great for breaking up long days of sitting at a desk, because the exercise strengthens and lengthens the muscles surrounding your shoulders.

1. **Get into a starting position of a push-up with your knees on the ground, as shown in Figure 4-11a.**

   Make yourself straight from your knees to your shoulders and position yourself so that your shoulders are directly over your wrists.

2. **Reach your left arm under your body to the right side, while keeping yourself straight from your knees to head, as shown in Figure 4-11b.**

   The shoulder of the supporting arm should be in retraction, meaning your chest should be as close to the ground as possible without bending your supporting arm.

3. **Then press the right arm into the ground and reach to the sky with the left arm, as shown in Figure 4-11c.**

   In this part of the movement, the right shoulder should be in protraction, meaning you should be making yourself as big as possible by pushing your shoulder away from your ear.

You can also do this exercise from a crawling position, which is a bit easier. Next time you're feeling a bit of discomfort from working at a desk, try doing just four repetitions on both sides. I bet you'll feel better!

Y cuffs

This is definitely a favorite for improving shoulder health and mobility, because it trains all the shoulder functions. In other words, a lot of commonly neglected functions are being trained with a beautifully simple movement.

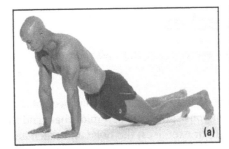

(a)

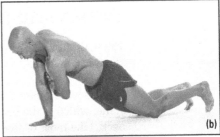

(b)

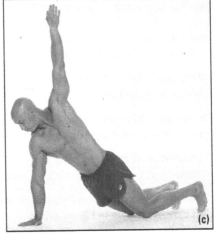

(c)

FIGURE 4-11:
The twist and
reach can
improve rotation
of the thoracic
spine and
shoulder mobility.

Photo by Jorge Alvarez, www.alvarezphoto.com

1. **Lie on your stomach with your arms at the Y position, thumbs up.**

   Make yourself as long as possible while looking down, but with your head off the ground, as shown in Figure 4-12a.

2. **Pull your hands under your armpits and reach toward your feet until your arms are straight, as shown in Figure 4-12b.**

   Work on keeping the rest of your body motionless as you do this.

3. **Place your hands on your lower back and let your elbows fall toward the ground, as shown in Figure 4-12c.**

4. **Raise your elbows as high as possible, as shown in Figure 4-12d.**

5. **Return your hands to your sides, as shown in Figure 4-12b, and then reverse the first part of the movement, pulling your hands through your armpits back to the starting position.**

For each portion of this exercise, challenge yourself to explore your full range of motion while keeping the rest of your body as long, straight, and motionless as possible.

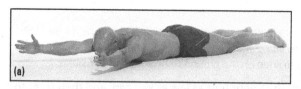

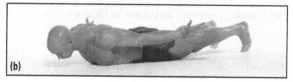

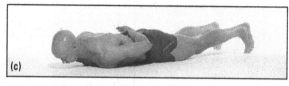

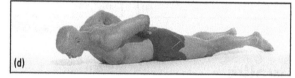

FIGURE 4-12:
The y cuffs
exercise improves
your shoulder
health and
mobility.

Photo by Jorge Alvarez, www.alvarezphoto.com

Side Lying Exercises

This movement selection focuses on the sides of your body to include the insides of your thighs. Here again, learn to make yourself long and straight. In a side planking or lying position, someone looking down on you should see a straight line. Push your hips forward by tightening your glutes, lift your chest slightly, tighten your midsection, and get your head into alignment.

Hip drops

The main purpose of this movements is to strengthen the sides of your body and improve side-to-side bending of the spine.

1. **Get into a long straight side planking position with your top leg in front of your bottom leg, as shown in Figure 4-13a.**

Make yourself as straight as possible by tightening your glutes and abs, while slightly lifting your chest. If this position proves too difficult, you can place your bottom knee on the ground to help hold the position.

2. **Slowly drop your hips as low as you can, and then reset to a straight and centered starting position, as shown in Figure 4-13b.**

FIGURE 4-13:
Hip drop starting position (a) and ending position (b).

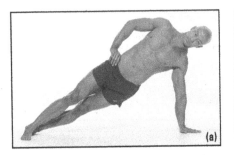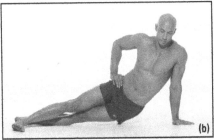

Photo by Jorge Alvarez, www.alvarezphoto.com

Moon walks

The main function of the moon walk is to work your hip abduction and adduction, which helps to move your legs toward and away from your body's center line.

1. **Get into a side planking position with your top foot in front of your bottom foot, as shown in Figure 4-14a.**

2. **Slide the bottom front in front of the top foot, and then place the top foot in front of the bottom foot.**

   You're essentially walking while in a side planking position (see Figure 4-14b).

3. **Walk forward four steps, and then walk backward four steps. See Figure 4-14c.**

You can also do this exercise while supporting yourself on the bottom forearm, instead of an extended arm. You can then use the top arm to support yourself by placing it on the ground in front of your stomach.

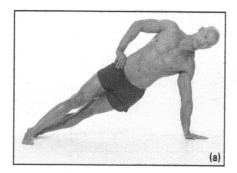
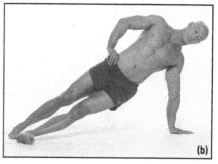
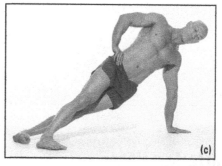

FIGURE 4-14: Get into a long straight side planking position with your top leg in front of your bottom leg (a), place the bottom leg in front of the top leg (b), and then place the top leg in front of the bottom leg (c).

Photo by Jorge Alvarez, www.alvarezphoto.com

Side crunches

The side crunch exercise strengthens the sides of your body and core with lateral flexion of the spine. This is a short movement that can feel a bit awkward at first, so be patient. Lateral stability is an often overlooked part of people's training program.

1. **Lie down on your left side with your legs elevated and your right hand on your head, as shown in Figure 4-15a.**

   Make yourself as straight as possible.

2. **While keeping your legs elevated and motionless, raise your right elbow and head with a short crunching movement, as shown in Figure 4-15b.**

For this short movement, ensure that the motion is coming from your midsection. Avoid pulling on your head.

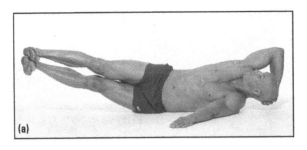

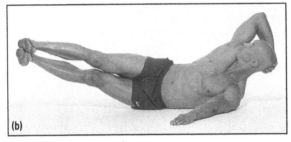

FIGURE 4-15:
Side crunch
starting position
(a) and ending
position (b).

Photo by Jorge Alvarez, www.alvarezphoto.com

Side leg lifts

This movement develops your upper glutes while teaching you to move your legs away from center line without externally rotating the hips. Learning to control hip rotation during hip abduction allows you to step laterally while keeping your knees and toes pointed straight ahead, which is typically safer and more efficient, like when playing tag with your kids.

As you do this exercise, keep your ankles flexed and toes pulled back toward your face. Your feet should remain parallel the entire time. The knee and toes of the elevated leg should never point up!

1. **Lay down on your left side with a long straight body position, as shown in Figure 4-16a.**

2. **While keeping the toes and knee of the elevated leg angled slightly down toward the ground (internally rotated), raise your right leg as high as you can, as shown in Figure 4-16b.**

The point of this exercise is to lift the top leg as high as possible without rotating your toes upward. If you're doing this movement correctly, you should feel the contraction in the upper glute of the elevated leg, and not in your hip flexor.

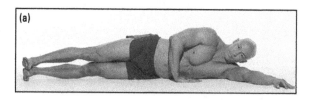

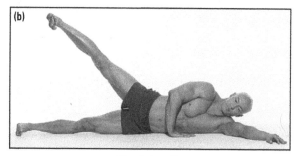

FIGURE 4-16:
Starting position (a) and ending position (b) for the side leg lift.

Photo by Jorge Alvarez, www.alvarezphoto.com

IN THIS CHAPTER

» Learning the rolling exercise

» Trying the lying to kneeling exercise

» Practicing the kneeling to standing exercise

» Learning the lying to stork stance exercise

Chapter **5**

Lying to Standing Transitions (Developmental Movements)

The essentials of athletic ability are learned early in life through *developmental movements*, which can be described as the movements needed to transition between lying, kneeling, and standing positions. Spinal stabilization, hip and shoulder coordination, and control of lateral weight shifting are the fundamentals on which locomotion is built.

Your performance with walking, running, throwing, striking, and many other activities depends on your mastery of these basics, and they are best improved by duplicating nature's learning process, which is a progression of transitions between lying, kneeling, and standing positions.

In this chapter, you're given a simple step-by-step guide to refining the skills you learned first in life.

WARNING

It's always a good idea to check with your doctor before you begin an exercise regimen. Also, if any of the exercises in this chapter cause you pain, stop doing them. It's important to be able to recognize the difference between something that is hard and something this is painful. No exercise should cause pain. Always listen to your body.

The Role of Weight Shifting in Movement and Stability

Weight shifting is one of those things that's so basic and common that most of us have never stopped to give it much thought or attention. However, control of weight shifting is so incredibly important, precisely because it's always in use. Every step you take involves a lateral weight shift, whether you're crawling, walking, jogging, or sprinting. Similarly, throwing a ball, swinging a club, or kicking a bag involve lateral weight shifts. Balance that is useful in real life expresses itself through improved control over rhythmic side-to-side weight shifting.

Exercises for Coordinating Hip and Shoulder Functions

Moving safely and effectively requires moving your arms and legs around a neutral spine. The floor exercises in Chapter 4 are a great way to learn that. The next step is to integrate your improved joint functions and posture into useful movements that involve weight shifting.

Rolling exercises

Rolling is the simplest example of coordinated hip and shoulder movement in order to create a lateral weight shift for the sake of getting from one place to another. With this simple exercise, you learn to move your arms around a neutral spine while shifting your weight laterally, which is also needed for much more complex movements, like sprinting and boxing.

1. **Lie on your back with your left arm extended past your head and your right arm perpendicular to your body, as shown in Figure 5-1a.**

2. **Initiate the roll by reaching across your body with your right arm while simultaneously crunching your abdominals slightly, as shown in Figure 5-1b.**

   The crunch and reach is needed to initiate the weight shift, so be sure to reach in the direction that you're trying to roll.

3. **Continue the roll until you're face down on the floor (see Figure 5-1c). Once you're in a front-lying position, place both your hands under your shoulders.**

   This small movement prepares you for transitions to other positions that you'll learn later.

4. **Reverse the movement by extending your left arm past your head, and then push off of your right hand to return to a back lying position.**

   In order to roll efficiently, you have to get your arm out of the way, which is also a great way to improve shoulder mobility.

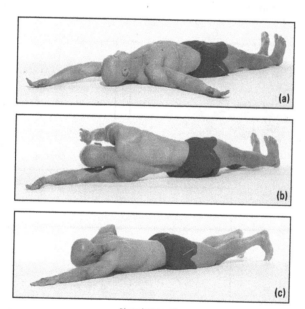

FIGURE 5-1: The rolling exercise.

Photo by Jorge Alvarez, www.alvarezphoto.com

Lying to kneeling exercises

This is a full-body movement that teaches you to transition smoothly from a front-lying position to a tall double-kneeling position. You'll develop useful strength while also improving your posture.

1. **Start from a front-lying position with your hands under your shoulders, as shown in Figure 5-2a.**

   If you have wrist pain, place you forearms on the ground with your elbows tucked in to your sides.

2. **Lift your hips and push them back as far as you can toward your heels (see Figure 5-2b).**

3. **Extend at your hips until you're in a tall, double-kneeling position, as shown in Figure 5-2c.**

   If you have knee pain or problems with your knees, try placing a pad under your knees.

4. **Reverse the movement by pushing your hips back, and then return to a front-lying position with both your hands under your shoulders.**

   Be sure to initiate the movement by pushing your hips back. That gives you much more control over the movement, so that you don't have to fall forward onto your hands.

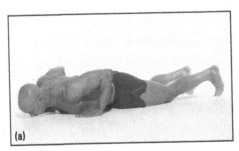
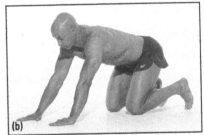
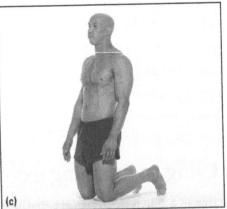

FIGURE 5-2:
The lying to kneeling exercise.

Photo by Jorge Alvarez, www.alvarezphoto.com

Kneeling to standing exercises

This exercise is exceptional for developing strength, flexibility, and balance that's useful in real life. As mentioned, almost everything you do in life involves stepping. As you do this exercise, work on taking big lunging steps while maintaining a tall, upright posture.

1. **From a tall, double-kneeling position, as shown in Figure 5-2c, shift your weight onto your right hip and bring your left foot forward, so that you end up in a single-kneeling position. See Figure 5-3a.**

   Feel free to use whatever arm position is comfortable for you. In these images, the arms are at the T position.

2. **Shift your weight onto your lead leg while pushing off your rear leg and move into a standing position. See Figure 5-3b.**

   Keep your midsection tight as you step forward. That helps keep your spine in a neutral position (meaning not unnecessarily arched), which is safest.

3. **Reverse the movement to get back to a double-kneeling position.**

   On the way down, maintain a tall upright posture with a tight midsection, and challenge yourself to take big steps.

FIGURE 5-3: Shift your weight onto your right hip and step forward into a single-kneeling position (a) and then move into a standing position with your arms out (b).

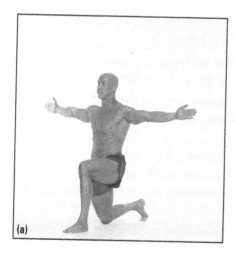 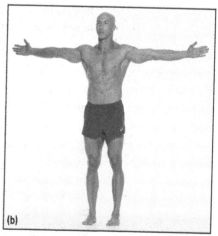

Photo by Jorge Alvarez, www.alvarezphoto.com

From lying to the stork stance exercises

This exercise combines all of the previous ones into one fluid movement. Once you feel confident in performing the previous exercises, you're ready to try this. Take your time and remember that practice makes you better!

REMEMBER

The point of these movements is to improve your balance, strength, and mobility in the most useful way possible, so that you can perform optimally, injury free. That requires you to prioritize your posture. For all these movements, lift your chest slightly while keeping your midsection tight, so that your spine is as long and straight as possible. It'll probably feel a bit awkward at first, but it'll soon become habitual, which is exactly what you want.

This exercise has all the benefits of the previous exercises, plus the additional challenge of a tall step-up position known as stork stance, as shown in Figure 5-4. The stork stance is a simple movement that has a big impact on athletic performance, because it improves your ability to take big steps while maintaining good posture.

1. **Follow the instructions in the "Rolling exercises" section to roll over.**

   From a back-lying position, roll left to a front-lying position, so that you are face-down with your hands under your shoulders.

2. **Push your hips back and lift your body to a tall, double-kneeling position, as shown previously in Figure 5-2c.**

3. **Step forward with the left leg to a single-kneeling position (as shown previously in Figure 5-3a), and then stand up.**

4. **Shift your weight right and lift your left knee while making yourself as tall and straight as possible.**

   This is called the *stork stance* and is shown in Figure 5-4. Prioritize standing up tall and straight on one leg. The height of your elevated knee is less important than your posture. In the beginning, it's okay to lift your knee off the ground just slightly. As your balance and mobility improve, gradually lift your knee higher and higher. Hold this position just long enough to get into the tallest possible position.

5. **Reverse the entire movement and return to a back-lying position.**

   As you transition from single-kneeling to stork stance, use whatever arm position is comfortable for you. In these images, the arms are at the T position.

You can do repeated repetitions on the same side before switching sides, or you can alternate sides after every rep.

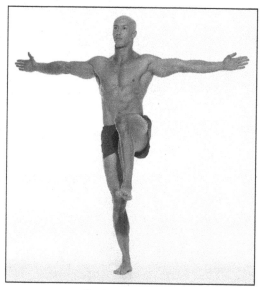

FIGURE 5-4:
The stork
stance improves
balance, posture,
and hip mobility

Photo by Jorge Alvarez, www.alvarezphoto.com

TIP

To make this exercise easier, move your arms freely. You can even push off the lead leg with one or both hands to assist the transition between single kneeling and standing.

TIP

Once you're familiar with this exercise and the movements are automatic, transition without stopping except briefly at the stork stance end position. But keep in mind that it's not about speed. Focus on making the movements as smooth and effortless as possible.

Chapter **6**

Strength Training Exercises for Your Core

The *core* refers to the muscles at the center of your body, which include your abdomen, lower back, hips, and pelvis. Strengthening these muscles improves posture by stabilizing your spine so you can maintain proper alignment for optimal force absorption. The benefits of a stable midsection include injury prevention, reduction of back pain, improved lifting, balance, stability, and better posture, as well as better athletic performance.

A strong core also forms the basis for generating power and transferring energy between the lower body and upper body, pain free.

WARNING It's always a good idea to check with your doctor before you begin an exercise regimen. Also, if any of the exercises in this chapter cause you pain, stop doing them. It's important to be able to recognize the difference between something that is hard and something this is painful. No exercise should cause pain. Always listen to your body.

Mastering the Abdominal Exercises

These exercises focus mainly on the rectus abdominis, which are the muscles that form your "six-pack." They also develop the transverse abdominis, obliques, hip flexors, and other supporting muscles. These movements are done mainly in planking and back lying positions, and their main function is developing the strength needed to resist unwanted movement through the midsection.

TIP

If you want detailed video tutorials for many of these exercises, go to the Instagram page *Mark_Lauren_Bodyweight*. You'll find a link in the bio that gives you access to all the free videos in the subscription app, *Mark Lauren On Demand*.

Bodyrocks

The bodyrock exercise involves moving forward and backward while holding a plank position. Try it by following these steps:

1. **Get in the starting position of a push-up and lower yourself down onto your forearms.**

   This called the *pillar* position.

   Your elbows should be slightly forward of your shoulders, and your hands should be shoulder-width apart, as shown in Figure 6-1a.

2. **From this position, move your body straight forward, rocking forward on your toes, as shown in Figure 6-1b, and then reset to the starting position.**

3. **Continue rocking back and forth while maintaining a perfectly straight body position from head to toes.**

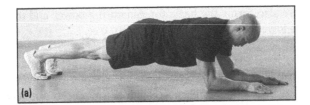

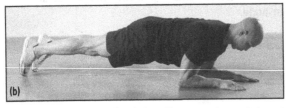

FIGURE 6-1: Get into a pillar position on your forearms (a) and then rock back and forth while keeping yourself straight (b).

Photo by Jorge Alvarez, www.alvarezphoto.com

REMEMBER

One of the most important parts of learning to move properly is learning how to make yourself long and straight. To get into ideal alignment, use the following checklist — flex your glutes, tighten your abs, lift your chest slightly, and get your head into alignment, so that your cervical spine is in a neutral position.

Reaching bodyrocks

Once you are able to perform regular bodyrocks with good form and relative ease, you can move on to reaching bodyrocks.

1. Get into the pillar position and rock your body backward as far as possible without lifting your hips, as shown in Figure 6-2a.

2. Rock forward, shift the weight of your upper body onto your right forearm, and reach as far forward as possible with your left arm, as shown in Figure 6-2b.

3. Return to the starting position and repeat with the opposite arm. Keep your body as straight and level throughout the movement as possible.

FIGURE 6-2: Start in a planking on your forearms (a) and then rock forward while reaching past your head with your left arm (b).

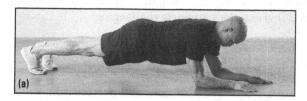

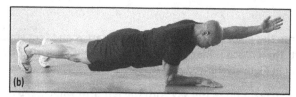

Photo by Jorge Alvarez, www.alvarezphoto.com

Side reaching bodyrocks

This variation of bodyrocks requires a lot of strength in order to prevent unwanted rotation. Make sure you're proficient with the first two bodyrock variations before trying this one.

1. Get in the pillar position with your feet shoulder-width apart.

2. Shift your weight onto your right forearm and then reach to the left as far as possible with your left arm, as shown in Figure 6-3.

3. Reset to the starting position and then switch sides.

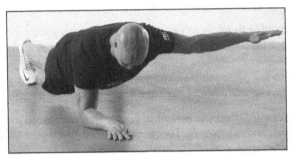

FIGURE 6-3: With the left arm, reach to your left side as far as possible. Then switch sides.

Photo by Jorge Alvarez, www.alvarezphoto.com

TIP

To get the full benefit of this exercise, be sure to shift your weight slightly in the direction you're reaching. This weight shift away from your center of gravity is what makes this exercise extremely challenging.

Pillar reaches

This exercise strengthens your core and posture while improving control of rotation.

1. Get into the pillar position with your forearms and feet shoulder-width apart. Then reach under your body to the right with your left arm, as shown in Figure 6-4a.

2. Reach straight up to the sky with the left arm while keeping your hips facing straight down at the ground, as shown in Figure 6-4b. Only open your chest!

3. Reset to the pillar position and then repeat on the other side.

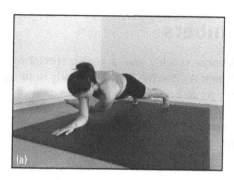
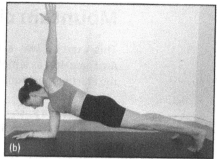

FIGURE 6-4:
This exercise
is great for
your core.

Photo courtesy of Lea Badenhoop

Tripod scissor kicks

This is a great movement for learning to control and resist rotation. The key is to keep your pelvis level as you perform this exercise. Take your time.

1. **Get into a the push-up position with your wrists directly under the shoulders. Place your feet shoulder-width apart or wider, and then lift the right foot a few inches off the floor, as shown in Figure 6-5a.**

2. **While keeping your toes and knees pointing straight down, bring your right foot to your left foot, as shown in Figure 6-5b. Reset to the starting position and switch sides.**

   The important part is to prevent unwanted movement as you lift the foot off the floor. Keep your spine, including your pelvis, stable.

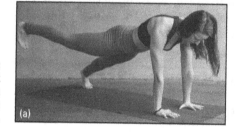
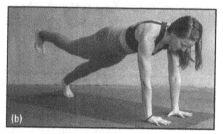

FIGURE 6-5:
Bring your right
leg to your left
and reset it to the
starting position.

Photo courtesy of Lea Badenhoop

The farther apart your feet are, the harder the exercise.

If you perform the exercise on your forearms, it will be easier on your arms but harder on your core.

TIP

Mountain climbers

This exercise was a favorite when I was a young special ops guy in the U.S. Air Force. It's as simple as it is effective. You're basically running in place while in the starting position of a push-up.

1. **Start in a push-up position, keeping your neck, spine, tailbone, and legs all in a straight line, as shown in Figure 6-6a.**

   Keep your arms straight with your wrists directly below your shoulders.

2. **Begin running in place by bringing your knees to your chest, as shown in Figure 6-6b.**

   Maintain a long straight body position and find a steady rhythm.

FIGURE 6-6:
Get into a high planking position (a) and run in place while keeping your hips low (b).

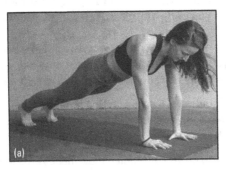 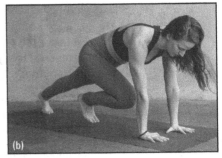

Photo courtesy of Lea Badenhoop

TIP

Your rear end may want to rise up as you bring your knees to your chest. Work on keeping your body parallel to the ground, even if it means limiting your knee movement when you first begin.

Mountain climbers across

This mountain climber variation develops your core and adductors, which are the muscles on the insides of your thighs.

1. **Get into the starting position of a push-up and then bring your right knee to your left elbow, as shown in Figure 6-7a.**

2. **Reset to the starting position and then bring your right knee to your left elbow, as shown in Figure 6-7b.**

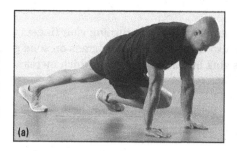
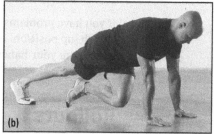

FIGURE 6-7:
From a push-up position, bring your right knee to your left elbow, then alternate knees.

This movement is not meant to be done quickly, like regular mountain climbers where you're running in place. Take your time and get a full range of motion while maintaining good form.

Mountain climbers around

This variation places more of an emphasis on the sides of your core. Again, take your time and challenge your range of motion with every rep.

1. **Get into the starting position of a push-up.**

2. **Shift your weight onto the left side of your body and then bring your right knee as close as possible to your right shoulder, as shown in Figure 6-8.**

For added difficulty, try doing this exercise from the pillar position.

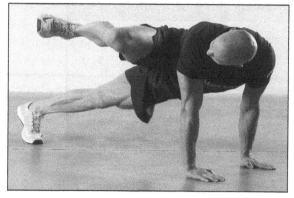

FIGURE 6-8:
From a plank, bring your right knee to your right shoulder.

TIP

If you have problems with wrist pain, try turning your fingers outward slightly in a push-up position. It also helps to place your hands on solid ground instead of a mat where your hands sink into a soft material, which increases the bend in your wrists.

Rollouts

This is an exceptional exercise for strengthening your midsection. It requires an ab roller or anything that allows you to slide, such as furniture sliders. There's plenty of room for creativity. You can also use magazines to slide on carpet or put socks on your hands to slide on tile and hardwood floors.

1. Get into a kneeling position with both knees on a padded surface and your hands on something that can slide (or roll), as shown in Figure 6-9a.

2. Flex your abdominals hard, tuck your tail bone, and then slide your hands away from your knees while keeping yourself straight from head to tailbone, as shown in Figure 6-9b.

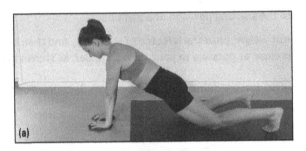

(a)

FIGURE 6-9:
Get to a kneeling position with your hands on something that can slide and move forward.

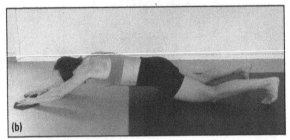

(b)

Photo courtesy of Lea Badenhoop

As you slide your hands forward, keep your hips off the ground as long as possible. For most people, this movement is more a controlled fall, which is okay. Simply do your best to control the descent. Once your hips are on the ground, continue to slide your hands forward as far as possible to make yourself long.

Cheat yourself back up to the starting position however you want, and then start again.

This exercise puts a fair amount of stress on your shoulders and midsection, so be sure to warm up thoroughly before trying it. Also, if you lack the strength and stability, bodyrocks can be used as an easier version of this exercise.

Hanging leg lifts

This is an exceptional core exercise that focuses on your lower abs and hip flexors, which are the muscles on the front of your thighs responsible for lifting your legs out in front of you. It's also great for strengthening your grip and improving shoulder health.

1. **Find something to hold onto and hang your entire body from it, as shown in Figure 6-10a.**

   It's best if it's high enough that your feet are off the ground when hanging. But if you can't find or reach something that high, it's okay to bend your knees in the starting position. I've used door frames, pull-up bars, tree limbs, the edge of a porch, and the top of a swing set, like in Figure 6-10a.

2. **While hanging, bring your knees up toward your chest until your knees are at least hip height, as shown in Figure 6-10b. Then lower them back down without swinging. Take the time to make yourself as straight as possible after every rep.**

If you want to add difficulty, you can keep your legs straight while bringing them up to your chest, as shown in Figure 6-11.

Scorpion kicks

This fun core movement improves hip, spine, and shoulder mobility.

1. **Get in the starting position of a push-up with your shoulders directly over your hands, as shown in Figure 6-12a.**

2. **Pull your right knee into your chest, as shown in Figure 6-12b.**

3. **Raise your right foot straight up into the air, as shown in Figure 6-12c, and continue across your body to the left side as far as possible, as shown in Figure 6-12d.**

   Think of your foot as a scorpion stinger that you're using to sting prey on the left side of you.

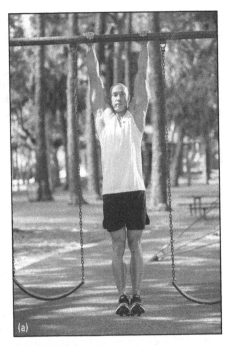

FIGURE 6-10:
Bring your knees up to your chest while hanging from something sturdy.

(a)

(b)

Photo by Jorge Alvarez, www.alvarezphoto.com

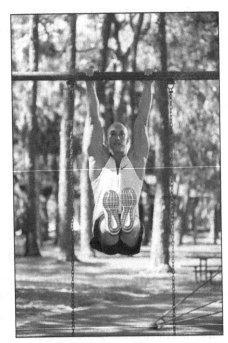

FIGURE 6-11:
Keep your legs straight for more difficulty.

Photo by Jorge Alvarez, www.alvarezphoto.com

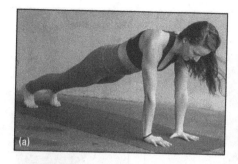
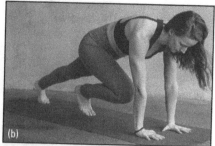
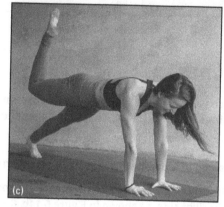
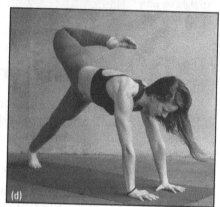

FIGURE 6-12:
The scorpion kick
improves hip,
spine, and
shoulder mobility.

Photo courtesy of Lea Badenhoop

Reset to the starting position and switch sides. An easier variation of this exercise is to reach the foot straight up toward the sky and then reset to switch sides.

Parallel leg crunches

The good ol' crunch! The crunch is different from a sit-up in that the movement focuses more on the abdominals and less on the hip flexors. In a sit-up, the bottom of the movement is engaging your abdominals, whereas the top of the movement engages the hip flexors. The crunch is basically the bottom half of a sit-up.

1. Lie down on your back with your arms reaching straight up to the sky and your hips, knees, and ankles bent at 90 degree angles, as shown in Figure 6-13a.

2. Without moving your legs, reach up as high as you can, as shown in Figure 6-13b.

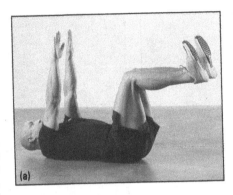
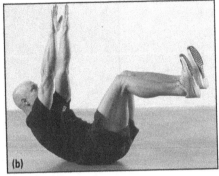

Photo by Jorge Alvarez, www.alvarezphoto.com

FIGURE 6-13:
Perform a
crunch and reach
straight up with
your arms.

Starfish crunches

This is my favorite crunch variation that I use to also improve control of hip rotation, so I can do basic things like walk and run with my knees and toes pointing in the right direction.

1. Start in the end position of a parallel leg crunch, as shown in Figure 6-14a.

2. Lower yourself while bringing your arms to the Y position and lowering your right leg to your right side, as shown in Figure 6-14b. Reset to the top of the movement and then repeat by lowering your right leg to your right side.

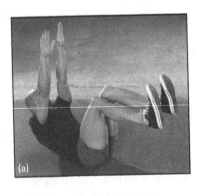
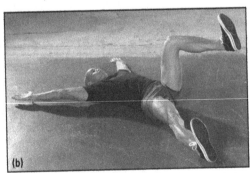

Photo by Jorge Alvarez, www.alvarezphoto.com

FIGURE 6-14:
Lower your arms
to the Y position
and extend one
leg to the side.

As you lower your legs, do your best to keep the knee and toes of the extended leg pointing straight up. You also want to make yourself as long as possible in the bottom position while flexing your abs.

Sit-ups

This is a classic core exercise that I did daily in the military.

1. **Lie on your back with your arms crossed and knees pointing up, as shown in Figure 6-15a.**

2. **While keeping your hips and feet on the ground, sit up until your torso is vertical, as shown in Figure 6-15b. Take a brief moment in the top position to make yourself straight by lifting your chest.**

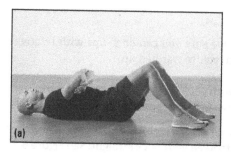 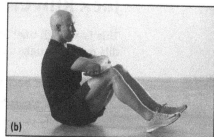

FIGURE 6-15: Starting position (a) and ending position (b) for sit-ups.

Photo by Jorge Alvarez, www.alvarezphoto.com

TIP

This exercise is significantly easier if you have someone pin your feet to the ground. Sliding your feet under a couch also works well, especially if there's a carpet to pad your tush. The tailbone can take a bit of beating with this exercise, especially if you do a lot of repetitions. In the military, we did hundreds of unassisted sit-ups on concrete, which was just plain mean.

V-ups

This is an excellent exercise for strengthening your abs and hip flexors while improving timing and coordination.

1. **Lie flat on your back with arms at your sides, as shown in Figure 6-16a.**

2. **While keeping only your butt on the ground, bring your chest and knees up toward each other until they almost touch, as shown in Figure 6-16b.**

Make yourself tall at the top of the movement by lifting your chest slightly. This movement requires a bit of timing and rhythm so don't get frustrated. Start by doing just a few reps at once to avoid fatigue. You'll learn faster that way.

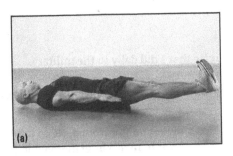 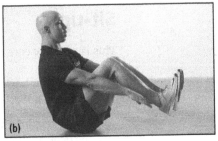

FIGURE 6-16:
V-ups
strengthening
your abs and
hip flexors.

Photo by Jorge Alvarez, www.alvarezphoto.com

Jack knives

This is a tough one! Make sure you can do v-ups with relative ease before trying this one, and make sure you're warmed up.

1. **Lie on your back with your feet elevated and your arms extended past your head, as shown in Figure 6-17a.**

2. **Forcefully swing your arms overhead and try to touch your toes while lifting your chest to keep your back straight. See Figure 6-17b.**

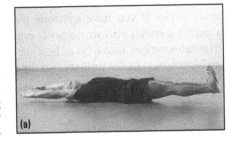 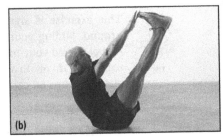

FIGURE 6-17:
Take a long,
straight starting
position for
jack knives.

Photo by Jorge Alvarez, www.alvarezphoto.com

A slightly harder variation of this exercise is to start this movement with your arms at your sides. From this position, you can't swing your arms, so your muscles will need to contract harder.

Practicing the Lateral Stability Exercises

These exercises strengthen the muscles responsible for controlling side-to-side movement and rotational forces, which translates to improved spinal alignment, athletic performance, and injury resistance.

Side plank

This simple exercise is a static hold that strengthens the sides of your body.

1. **Get to a push-up position and then lower yourself onto your forearms (into the pillar position).**

2. **Shift your weight onto your left side and rotate until you are in a side planking position, as shown in Figure 6-18.**

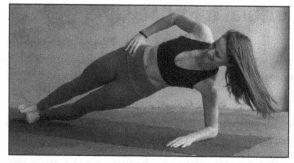

FIGURE 6-18:
Hold this static position, while making yourself long and straight.

Photo courtesy of Lea Badenhoop

Start with short, repeated holds of just 15 seconds, so you can focus on getting into correct alignment. Rest as much as you need. You'll make solid progress from being consistent. You don't need to kill yourself. Enjoy!

REMEMBER

A basic and very important skill is being able to make yourself long and straight. You'll want to be able to do this in all different situations, which is why you practice this in back lying positions, pillar positions, side planking and so on. To make yourself straight, use the following checklist of cues — flex your glutes, tighten your abs, lift your chest, and get your head into position, so that your entire body is straight head to heels.

Side v-ups

This movement is great for developing the sides of your core!

1. **Lie on your right side with your legs straight and slightly off the ground, as shown in Figure 6-19a. Make yourself long and straight.**

2. **Press your bottom arm into the ground and bring your left elbow to your knees, as shown in Figure 6-19b.**

Just like regular v-ups, this exercise requires some timing and rhythm, so be patient with yourself and start with plenty of easy practice.

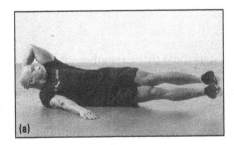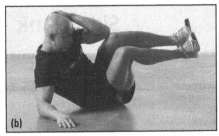

FIGURE 6:19: The side v-up starting position (a) and ending position (b).

Photo by Jorge Alvarez, www.alvarezphoto.com

ITB (Iliotibial band) leg lifts

This is an excellent mobility exercise that strengthens the muscles on the insides of your thighs, which are used for hip adduction and internal hip rotation. I often use this exercise as a warm up to avoid extremely annoying injuries, such as a pulled groin.

1. **Lie on your side with your top leg crossed over your bottom leg, as shown in Figure 6-20a.**

   You can grab the ankle of your top leg with your top arm to help you maintain a comfortable position.

2. **Fully rotate the knee of the bottom leg up toward the sky and then lift the leg as high as you can, as shown in Figure 6-20b.**

   Lower the leg while maintaining internal hip rotation and repeat.

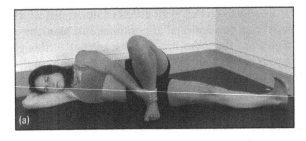

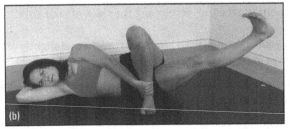

FIGURE 6-20: The starting position (a) and ending position (b) for ITB Leg Lifts.

Photo courtesy of Lea Badenhoop

ITB kickouts

This is a tough exercise that requires a pretty good amount of flexibility. The main focus for this exercise is strengthening the insides of your thighs.

1. **Get into a push-up position with your feet hip-width apart, as shown in Figure 6-21a.**

2. **Roll onto the inside of your right foot and bring the left knee to the right elbow. Then fully extend the left leg, as shown in Figure 6-21b.**

   As much as possible, try to point your left knee up toward the sky while extending the leg. It's super hard . . . just do the best you can! Reset to the starting position and switch sides.

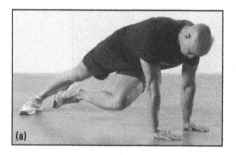 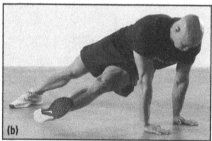

FIGURE 6-21: ITB kickouts are advanced exercises for your thighs.

Photo by Jorge Alvarez, www.alvarezphoto.com

For an easier variation of this exercise, bring your knee to your opposite elbow without extending the leg. It's just like doing mountain climbers across except that you're also rolling onto the inside of the supporting foot.

Learning the Lower Back Exercises

A strong lower back is an essential part of having a strong core. While the lower back is effectively developed with leg exercises, such as squats and side lunges, it's still a good idea to further strengthen them with more isolated movements. Combining these lower back exercises with leg exercises is an excellent way to improve your technique and functional strength.

Reverse hypers

We all need a strong backside to avoid injuries and lower back pain. This exercise is second to none for that purpose.

1. **Lie on a sturdy counter top, table, or park bench with your legs hanging off, as shown in Figure 6-22a.**

2. **While holding on to the supporting surface with your arms, fully straighten your legs, as shown in Figure 6-22b.**

   Lift your legs in a slow, controlled motion. Don't swing them. As always, make yourself as long and straight as possible.

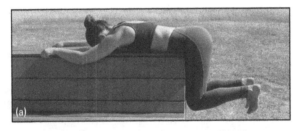

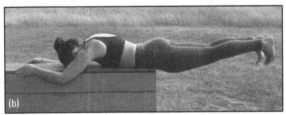

FIGURE 6-22: The starting position (a) and ending position (b) for reverse hypers.

Photo courtesy of Lea Badenhoop

You can make this exercise easier by doing just one leg at a time. To work your glutes more, spread your legs on the way up and hold a one- to three second pause before lowering your legs.

Swimmers

These days, we spend an incredible amount of time sitting in chairs with our arms in front of us, just as I am now while writing this. To break up too many hours of sitting, use swimmers to wake you up and activate all the dormant muscles of your backside.

1. Lie flat on your stomach with your arms extended past your head, as shown in Figure 6-23a.

2. Lift your right leg and left arm, as shown in Figure 6-23b, and then switch sides.

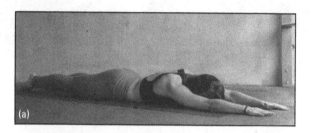

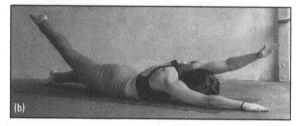

FIGURE 6-23: Raise the right leg and left arm and then switch.

Photo courtesy of Lea Badenhoop

Don't worry if you have a very limited range of motion with this exercise. People often see progress after just a single set. With regular practice, you'll be sitting, standing, and walking straighter.

Skydivers

Skydivers open your chest and strengthen your back, while seriously firing up your glutes.

1. Lie on your stomach with your legs spread wider than shoulder-width apart and your arms at the T position, as shown in Figure 6-24a. Your head, arms, and feet should be off the ground.

2. Without moving your upper body, close your legs, as shown in Figure 6-24b. Continue by rhythmically opening and closing your legs.

You can also do this exercise by holding your arms at your sides (easier) or by holding your arms at the Y position (harder).

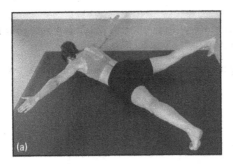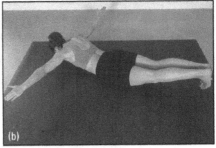

FIGURE 6-24:
Starting
position (a) and
ending position (b)
for skydivers.

Photo courtesy of Lea Badenhoop

Chapter **7**

Strength Training Exercises for Your Legs and Hips

The leg and hip exercises in this chapter will provide you with the strength, flexibility, balance, and coordination needed to move through life with full confidence. When they are done correctly, these movements develop stability and mobility throughout your entire body. Classic exercises, such as squats and lunges, are taught in a way that ensure you get the best possible transfer of improved performance from your workouts to real life and sports.

WARNING

It's always a good idea to check with your doctor before you begin an exercise regimen. Also, if any of the exercises in this chapter cause you pain, stop doing them. It's important to be able to recognize the difference between something that is hard and something this is painful. No exercise should cause pain. Always listen to your body.

Trying the Hip Hinging Exercises

Athletic performance, injury resistance, and general aesthetics are highly dependent on the strength and health of your hips. The main way that your body absorbs, transfers, and generates force is through hip hinging, which involves bending at the hips while maintaining a neutral spine. Examples of hip hinging include squatting, bending, lunging, and jumping.

If you want to develop a strong, healthy body that moves effectively in day-to-day life and sports, you need to learn to hip hinge while following a few basic rules that you can apply to all of the exercises in this chapter:

>> **Keep your feet parallel.** That means your toes should always point straight ahead, not outward or inward.

>> **Point your knees straight ahead.** You want your knees pointing in the same direction as your toes, meaning straight ahead. You have to learn to control hip rotation!

>> **Move your hips back.** Initiate hip hinging movements by pushing your hips back, as if you're bumping someone standing too close behind you.

>> **Lift your chest.** Keep your midsection tight and lift your chest slightly.

You're going to hear these coaching cues repeatedly throughout this chapter, because they apply to all exercises. Keeping your knees and toes pointing straight ahead, pushing your hips back, and maintaining a neutral spine ensures that your training develops postural habits that make you more efficient and injury resistant when you're not exercising.

Deadlifts

The bodyweight deadlift is a movement that teaches you to bend forward with optimal mechanics, which involves pushing your hips back and keeping your back straight, which can take a bit of practice. It helps to have a mirror for this exercise, so you can see what your back is doing.

1. Get into the starting position, as shown in Figure 7-1a, with your feet hip-width apart and your arms overhead in the streamline position, as if you're diving into a pool.

2. **Push your hips back and bend forward with the knees slightly bent, as shown in Figure 7-1b.**

   Keep your midsection tight and your back flat. Only go as far down as you can while maintaining a neutral spine. Your feet should remain parallel with your knees facing forward.

TIP

If you have problems keeping your back straight, place your hands on your knees in the bottom position of a deadlift. Then straighten your back. Once your back is straight, take your hands off your knees and complete the rep.

FIGURE 7-1:
Deadlifts are a bending exercise with your knees bent.

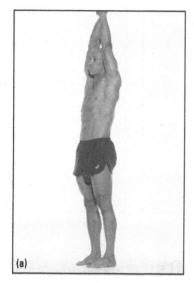

(a)   (b)

Photo by Jorge Alvarez, www.alvarezphoto.com

REMEMBER

For all the starting and ending positions in this section, stand up as straight as possible. Your feet should be parallel, your glutes flexed, your midsection tight, and your chest up. After every rep, be sure that you're standing up straight!

One-legged deadlifts

These are just like regular deadlifts except that you're doing them with one leg at a time to further improve strength and balance.

1. **Start with your feet hip-width apart and parallel. Bring your arms overhead to the streamline position.**

2. **Shift your weight onto your left leg and then pick up your right foot behind yourself, as shown in Figure 7-2a.**

3. Push your hips straight back while raising your right leg behind and bend forward with the upper body while keeping your spine long and neutral, as shown in Figure 7-2b.

4. Your toes of your supporting foot should face straight ahead. Reset to a standing position, and then switch sides.

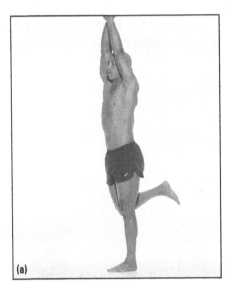 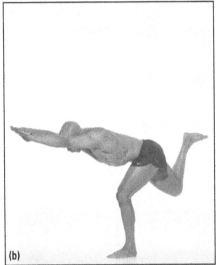

FIGURE 7-2:
Stand on one leg with your arms overhead (a) and then push your hips back and bend forward (b).

(a) (b)

Photo by Jorge Alvarez, www.alvarezphoto.com

Romanian deadlifts

This is an exceptional exercise that lengthens and strengthens your entire body, head to heels, especially the hamstrings.

1. Stand with your feet hip-width apart and arms overhead, as shown in Figure 7-3a.

2. With your legs straight, push your hips back while bending forward with a neutral spine, as shown in Figure 7-3b.

3. Bend forward until you feel a stretch in your hamstrings. Go only as far as you can without rounding the back! That means keep your spine in a neutral position.

Before reversing the movement, take a moment to make yourself as long and straight as possible while keeping your midsection tight.

If you can only bend forward slightly before you feel your hamstrings engage, don't worry. Just keep going as far as you can without rounding your back, and with enough repetition, your entire backside will become stronger and more flexible.

FIGURE 7-3:
Push your hips back and bend forward while keeping your legs and back straight.

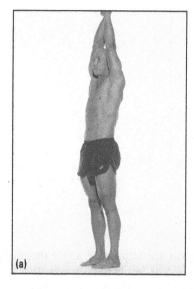

(a)

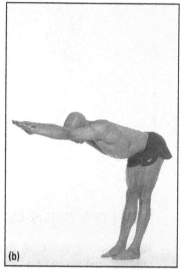

(b)

Photo by Jorge Alvarez, www.alvarezphoto.com

One-legged Romanian deadlifts

As the name implies, this is the one-legged version of Romanian deadlifts. It further challenges your balance and strength. Before attempting this version, it is advisable to first master regular two-legged deadlifts.

1. **Get into a standing position, as shown in Figure 7-4a, with your arms at the streamline position and your right foot slightly off the ground.**

2. **With the toes of your supporting foot pointing straight ahead, bring your right leg behind yourself while hinging forward with the upper body, as shown in Figure 7-4b.**

    Keep the knee of your elevated leg pointing straight down at the ground and maintain a straight line from the heel of the elevated leg to the head. Reverse the motion once you feel a good stretch in the hamstring of the supporting leg. Switch legs after reach repetition.

Throughout the movement, make yourself as long as possible. Lift the elevated leg behind yourself as high as you can while fully straightening your arms and legs.

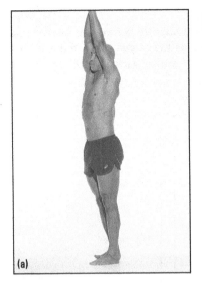
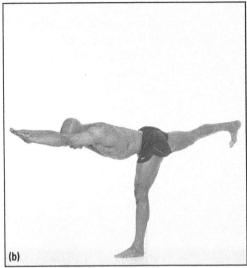

FIGURE 7-4:
Bend forward
while lifting your
right leg behind.

(a) (b)

Photo by Jorge Alvarez, www.alvarezphoto.com

Narrow squats

This squatting variation is great for improving ankle mobility, controlling hip rotation, and correcting posture. The key is to keep your toes and knees pointing straight and your chest up, especially in the bottom position.

1. **Stand with your feet hip-width apart and your arms in front of you, as shown in Figure 7-5a.**

2. **Push your hips back bend your knees as if you're sitting onto a chair, as shown in Figure 7-5b.**

   As you sit back, lift your chest up and keep your toes and knees pointing straight ahead. Challenge yourself to go as deep as you can while maintaining correct alignment. Then stand up straight before repeating.

TIP

When you first start doing this movement, it's not a bad idea to sit onto an actual chair. Sitting onto a chair gets you to push your hips back. When first learning to squat, people often sink their hips straight down, which puts the knees and ankles in vulnerable positions.

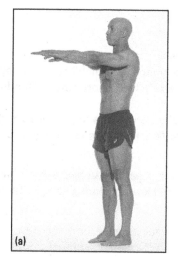 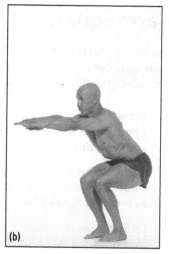

FIGURE 7-5:
Push your hips
back and down as
if sitting onto
a chair.

Photo by Jorge Alvarez, www.alvarezphoto.com

Wide squats

For this squatting variation, your feet are slightly wider than shoulder-width
apart. This places more emphasis on hip mobility and glute activation.

1. Stand with your feet shoulder-width apart and your arms in front of you,
    as shown in Figure 7-6a. Position your feet so that your toes are pointing
    straight ahead.

2. Push your hips back and sink your hips down while lifting your chest and
    keeping your knees pointing straight ahead, as shown in Figure 7-6b.

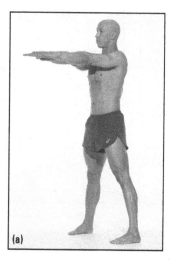 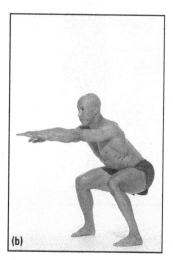

FIGURE 7-6:
Push your hips
back and down
while keeping
your back
straight.

Photo by Jorge Alvarez, www.alvarezphoto.com

T-arm squats

Performing squats with your arms at the T position strengthens your upper back, opens your chest, and challenges your ankle mobility. They key is to maintain alignment even if it means using a relatively short range of motion.

1. **Stand with your feet shoulder-width apart and your arms at the T position, as shown in Figure 7-7a. Fully extend through your arms and fingertips.**

2. **Push your hips back, bend your knees and sit back while lifting your chest and keeping your toes and knees pointing straight ahead, as shown in Figure 7-7b.**

   Go as deep as you can while maintaining good form. Then reverse the movement.

After every rep, stand up straight, check the position of your feet and arms, and then go again.

TIP

You can make all the squatting, bending, and lunging exercises harder or easier by varying the arm positions, and it's worth playing around with different options. In order of increasing difficulty, the main arm positions are as follows: arms front, arms at T, hands behind head, and arms at streamline.

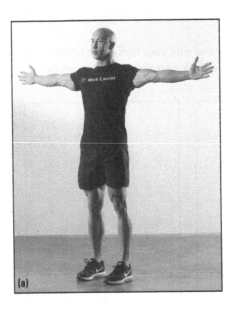
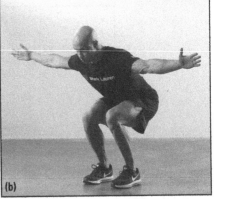

FIGURE 7-7: Push your hips back and down while lifting your chest.

Photo by Jorge Alvarez, www.alvarezphoto.com

(a)

(b)

Overhead squats

This squatting variation requires a quite a lot of ankle, hip, and shoulder mobility. But don't worry — simply do what you can and improve your range of motion gradually with consistent practice.

1. **Stand with your feet shoulder-width apart and place your arms at the Y position with a towel or broom held overhead slightly wider than shoulder-width apart. See Figure 7-8a.**

2. **Sink into a squat while doing your best to hold your towel directly over the midpoint of your feet, as shown in Figure 7-8b. Stand up after every rep.**

To make this squatting variation a bit easier, you can rotate your knees outward while in the bottom position. It also helps to be warmed up properly!

FIGURE 7-8: Squat down while keeping your arms extended overhead.

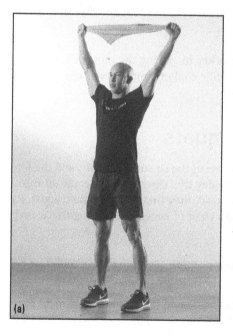 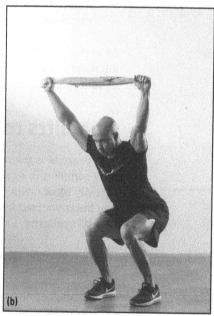

Photo by Jorge Alvarez, www.alvarezphoto.com

Squats to deadlifts

This movement is a T-arm squat with a transition from the bottom of the squat to the bottom of a Romanian deadlift with your arms at the streamline position. Performing this transition will strengthen and lengthen your entire body, while developing valuable postural habits.

1. Get into the starting position of a T-arm squat with your feet parallel and hip-width apart, as shown in Figure 7-9a.

2. Push your hips back and down while keeping your chest up,. Then get into the bottom of a T-arm squat, as shown in Figure 7-9b.

3. Straighten your legs and reach past your head while keeping your back straight. Get into the bottom of a streamline Romanian deadlift, as shown in Figure 7-9c.

4. Return to the bottom of a T-arm squat and then stand up straight to complete the rep.

As with all exercises, the key to getting the most out of this exercise is to stay in alignment at all times while challenging yourself to get every last millimeter out of your range of motion.

Deadlifts to squats

This exercise is the reverse of the squat to deadlift, and the hip hinging pattern is very common in day-to-day life. Often, when people sit into a chair, they don't actually squat down. Instead, they first bend and then squat. Pay attention to how you lower yourself into a chair or couch after trying this exercise to see if you can see the similarity.

1. Get into the starting position of a Romanian deadlift, as shown in Figure 7-10a.

2. Push your hips back and bend forward with a straight back until you feel a strong stretch in your hamstrings, as shown in Figure 7-10b.

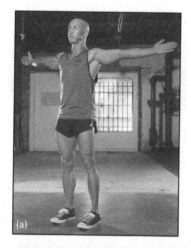
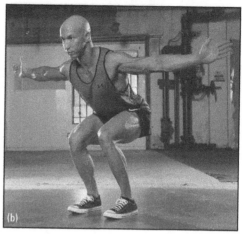

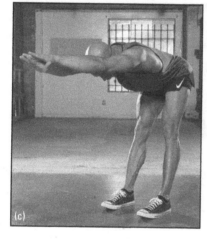

FIGURE 7-9:
Straighten your legs, bend forward, and reach to the streamline position.

Photo by Jorge Alvarez, www.alvarezphoto.com

3. **Transition to the bottom of a T-arm squat, as shown in Figure 7-10c.**

4. **Reset to the bottom of a Romanian deadlift with your arms at the streamline position, and then stand up straight to complete the repetition.**

Remember to keep your arms straight as you transition between the streamline Romanian deadlift and the T-arm squat.

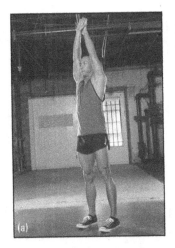
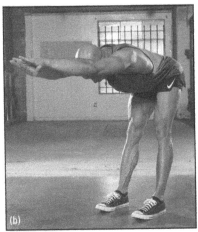
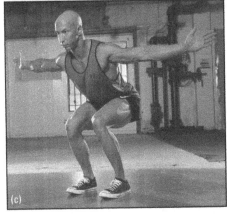

FIGURE 7-10:
Fully extend
through your
fingertips as if
lightning bolts
were coming out
of them.

Photo by Jorge Alvarez, www.alvarezphoto.com

One-legged squats

This movement is most similar to the narrow squat, but obviously you're squatting with just one leg.

1. While standing in front of a chair, as shown in Figure 7-11a, lift your right foot in front of yourself and stand on your left leg with your arms extended in front, zombie style.

2. Slowly lower your body by bending your left knee and pushing your hips back.

3. **With your back straight, sit onto the chair in a controlled manner without "flopping." See Figure 7-11b.**

   Once your butt is on the chair, rock your upper body back slightly and then use the forward momentum of your upper body rocking forward to help you stand up.

To make this exercise easier, stand in front of a door way with a chair behind you, so you can place your hands on the inside of the doorway for assistance.

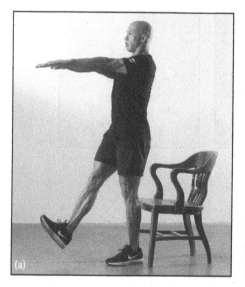 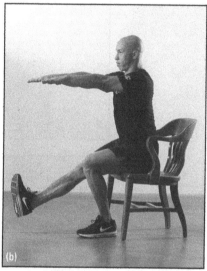

FIGURE 7-11: The one-legged squat starting position in front of a chair.

Photo by Jorge Alvarez, www.alvarezphoto.com

Squat thrusts

This is an athletic movement that requires timing, strength, and flexibility. As the Navy SEALs say, slow is smooth, and smooth is fast!

1. **Get into a squatting position with your feet hip- to shoulder-width apart and parallel. Your knees should point straight ahead with your hips back and your chest up, as shown in Figure 7-12a.**

2. **Place your hands on the ground in front of your feet, as shown in Figure 7-12b.**

3. **Jump your feet back to the starting position of a push-up, as shown in Figure 7-12c.**

4. In one fluid movement, pop back up to the squatting position with your feet and knees pointing straight ahead, hips back, and chest up.

The squat should look and feel like an athletic ready position from which you could instantly jump, sprint, or catch a ball.

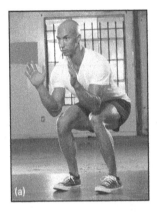 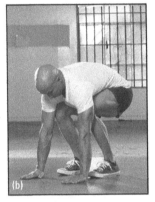

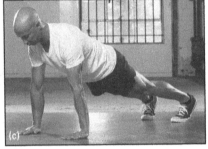

FIGURE 7-12: The squat thrust requires timing, strength, and flexibility.

Photo by Jorge Alvarez, www.alvarezphoto.com

Bulgarian split squats

This leg exercise seriously strengthens your thighs and hips while also stretching your hip flexors, which can become tight from sitting too much.

1. Place your right leg on a knee height object, such as a chair or coffee table, that's about one normal step behind you.

2. Bring your arms overhead to the streamline position, as shown in Figure 7-13a, and tighten your abdominals as if someone might punch you in the gut.

3. Sink your hips back and down as far as you can while keeping your torso upright and your midsection tight, as shown in Figure 7-13b.

For comfort, you can put a pillow on the chair and your foot on the pillow. Work on your balance and don't hold onto anything. This is a great exercise that works both legs, but be sure to push mainly off the foot that is on the ground. This is also a great way to lead up to doing one-legged squats.

TIP

You can make this exercise easier by holding your arms to the front, in the zombie position. Placing your arms at the T position or your hands behind head are also great options. Mix it up!

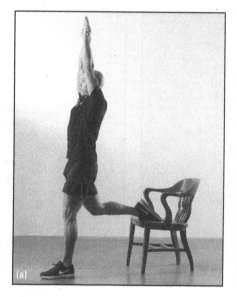
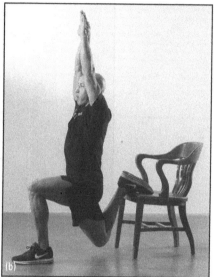

FIGURE 7-13: For Bulgarian split squats, sink your hips back and down.

Photo by Jorge Alvarez, www.alvarezphoto.com

Dynamic squats

This is a fun exercise that really burns and builds your backside. Stay relaxed and find a good rhythm.

1. **Start in a standing position with your feet hip-width apart and your hands at your sides, as shown in Figure 7-14a.**

2. **With a slight hop, jump your feet out to wider than shoulder-width apart and immediately push your hips back and try to touch the ground between your legs. Keep your back flat, as shown in Figure 7-14b.**

3. **Pop back up with another slight jump to return to the starting position.**

The rhythm for this exercise is similar to doing jumping jacks. Stay relaxed and light on your feet as you jump in and out of the starting and ending positions. Ensure that your toes and knees are pointing in the same direction (straight ahead).

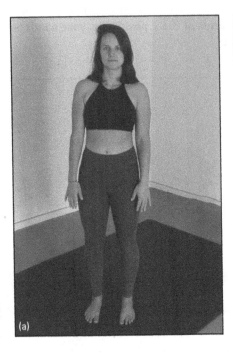 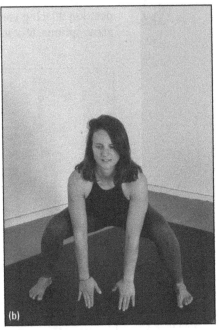

FIGURE 7-14: Starting position (a) and ending position (b) for dynamic squats.

Photo courtesy of Lea Badenhoop

Learning the Lunging Exercises

Lunges are basically giant steps that can be done in all directions — forward, backward, and laterally. All lunges involve a one-legged hip hinge as well a lateral weight shift, which is why they are an incredible tool for improving strength and balance. No other set of exercises will make you more sure on your feet than lunging movements.

As with all exercises, the accuracy of your technique will determine the safety of the movement. Make sure that you're warmed up properly and focused on your form. Your toes and knees should face in the same direction, which for lunging is either straight ahead or straight down.

Back lunges

The back lunge is the best way to learn lunging movements, because stepping to the rear automatically pulls your hip backward and away from your feet, which puts you into better alignment to safely absorb the force.

1. **Stand with your feet hip-width apart and your arms in the streamline position, as shown in Figure 7-15a.**

2. **Take a big step backward and lower your hips until your trailing knee almost touches the ground, as shown in Figure 7-15b.**

   Keep your midsection tight and your torso vertical! Return to the starting position and switch sides.

You can make this exercise easier by holding your arms to the front or at the T position.

REMEMBER

Before you sink into the bottom of a lunge, especially a long lunging position, flex your abdominals as if you're about to get punched in the gut. That'll help keep your spine in a neutral position. Most people have tight hip flexors, which cause them to arch through the back in deep lunging positions. To improve the flexibility of your hip flexors and stay in better posture, tighten your abs.

FIGURE 7-15: Stand with your arms in the streamline position (a) and then step backward while maintaining an upright torso (b).

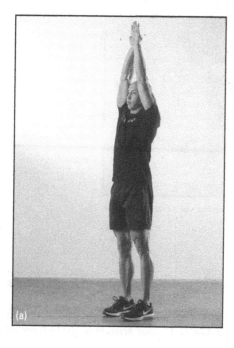
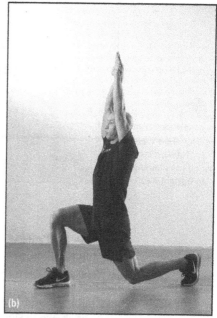

(a)　　　　(b)

Photo by Jorge Alvarez, www.alvarezphoto.com

Front lunges

Once you can do back lunges with good form, you're ready to move on to forward lunges.

1. **Stand with your feet hip-width apart. You can use any arm position.**

2. **Take a big step forward and sink your hips straight down as soon as the lead foot touches the ground. Maintain a tight midsection and an upright torso. See Figure 7-16.**

3. **Push off the lead leg and return to the starting position.**

The key to performing this exercise correctly is to sink the hips straight down as soon as the lead foot touches the ground. Avoid letting the forward momentum of your step carry your knee past your lead foot. In the end position, the lead knee should be directly above the lead foot.

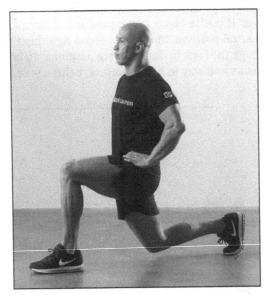

FIGURE 7-16:
Take a big forward step while maintaining an upright torso.

Photo by Jorge Alvarez, www.alvarezphoto.com

Side lunges

Side lunges are the next step in the progression of lunge exercises.

1. **Stand upright with your feet pointing straight ahead and hip-width apart, as shown in Figure 7-17a. Hold your arms straight in front of your body.**

2. **Take a wide step to the right with your right foot, as shown in Figure 7-17b.**

   As your right foot comes in contact with the ground, shift your weight onto it and push your hips back while lifting your chest. Your toes and knee of your right leg should remain facing straight ahead. Push off your right leg to return to the starting position, and then switch sides.

TIP

To make this exercise easier, perform this movement without stepping. Start with your feet significantly wider than shoulder-width apart. Shift your weight onto your right leg by pushing your hips back, bending your right leg and straightening your left leg. Shift your weight left in the same manner, and then continue to switch side to side.

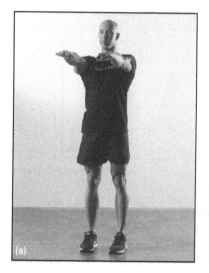 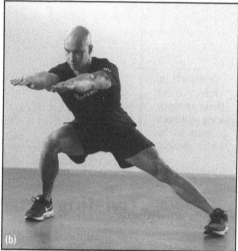

FIGURE 7-17:
Push your hips back and lift your chest up.

Photo by Jorge Alvarez, www.alvarezphoto.com

Saxon lunges

This is an incredible mobility exercise that requires a good amount of strength and stability. You can make this movement easier by placing the trailing knee on the ground.

1. **From a standing position with your arms in the streamline position, step back into a deep back lunge, as shown in Figure 7-18a.**

2. **While keeping your trailing knee pointing straight down at the ground and your arms straight, bend to the side of the forward leg, as shown in Figure 7-18b.**

3. Now bend to the opposite side, as shown in Figure 7-18c, while keeping your elbows straight, head in line with your spine, and abdominals tight.

4. Return to the middle and then stand up straight before switching sides.

To make this exercise a bit easier, tilt just to the side of the lead leg before returning to the starting position.

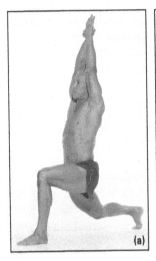 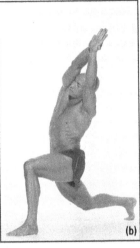 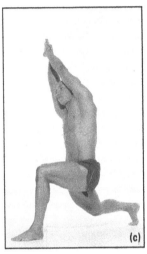

FIGURE 7-18: You can make these easier by placing your back knee on the ground.

(a)   (b)   (c)

Photo by Jorge Alvarez, www.alvarezphoto.com

Twisting lunges

This movement is similar to the Saxon lunge except that you're twisting in the bottom of a lunge instead of tilting. Again, you can make this exercise easier by resting your trailing knee on the ground.

1. Step into a back lunge with your arms at the streamline position, as shown in Figure 7-19a. Keep your abdominals tight to avoid arching through your back.

2. Twist to the side of the lead leg, as shown in Figure 7-19b, by pulling your left shoulder blade back.

3. Return to the middle and then stand up. Switch sides.

You can make this exercise a bit harder by twisting to both sides while holding the bottom of a lunge.

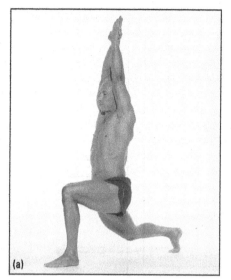 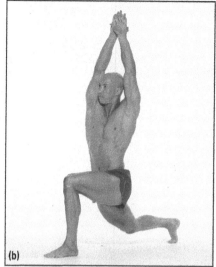

FIGURE 7-19: Step into a streamline back lunge (a) and then twist to the side of the lead leg (b).

Squats to lunges

The transition from squats to lunges is an excellent way to develop the strength, balance, and postural habits needed for more difficult exercises, such as one-legged squats.

1. **Stand up straight with your feet hip-width apart and your toes pointing straight head, as shown in Figure 7-20a. Hold your arms straight out in front of your body.**

2. **Push your hips back and sink into the bottom of a squat, as shown in Figure 7-20b. Keep your chest up and knees pointing straight ahead.**

3. **Shift your weight onto your left leg, and then step back with your right leg into the bottom of a lunge.**

   Your trailing knee should be on the ground, as shown in Figure 7-20c.

4. **While keeping your hips low and chest up, return to the bottom of a squat, and then stand up.**

   For the next rep, step back with your left leg.

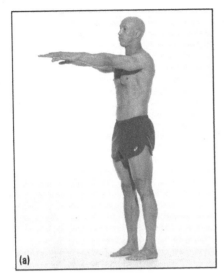

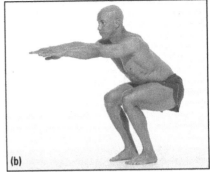

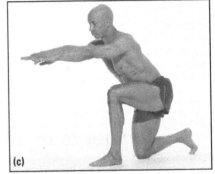

FIGURE 7-20: Try different arm positions to change the difficulty of this movement.

Photo by Jorge Alvarez, www.alvarezphoto.com

Lunges to squats

This is the reverse of the squat to lunge.

1. Stand up straight with your feet hip-width apart and your toes pointing straight head, as shown in Figure 7-21a. Hold your arms straight out in front.

2. Step back with your right leg into a single kneeling position, as shown in Figure 7-21b.

3. Shift your weight fully onto your left leg, push your hips back, and climb into the bottom of a squat while keeping your hips low and your chest up, as shown in Figure 7-21c.

4. Stand up straight and then step back with your left leg.

The transition from a single kneeling position to a deep squatting position is a good way to improve controlled weight shifting as well as the postural habits needed for good squatting technique. As you transition from single kneeling to squatting, keep your hips low and your chest up.

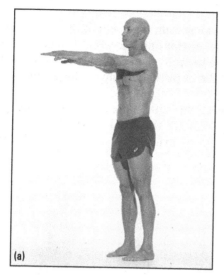

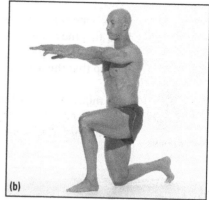

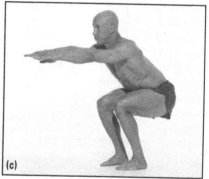

Photo by Jorge Alvarez, www.alvarezphoto.com

FIGURE 7-21:
This exercise
is a good way
to improve
controlled
weight shifting.

Iron Mikes

Once you've mastered all previous lunging exercises, you'll be ready for iron mikes. This exercise develops serious strength, and it should only be done when you are fresh, yet warmed up. It's best to keep the total number of reps low and take breaks.

1. Get in the bottom position of a back lunge, with your left leg forward, an upright torso, and your lead knee directly over (not in front of) your lead ankle, as shown in Figure 7-22a.

2. From this position, jump into the air and immediately switch the positions of your legs, as shown in Figure 7-22b, so that you land in the bottom of a lunge with your right leg forward, as shown in Figure 7-22c.

3. Maintain an upright torso and ensure that your lead knee is directly above your lead ankle when you land.

    As you make contact with the ground, immediately sink into the bottom of the next lunge and repeat.

If it's done correctly, with an upright torso and the hips back relative to the lead foot, this movement safely develops high levels of balance, speed, coordination, endurance, and power. The key is to plant the lead foot far enough in front of the hips so that the lead heel can be planted firmly on the ground.

WARNING

Iron mikes are high impact. Strength and correct positioning are important to safely absorb the force. Don't try these unless regular lunging exercises have become easy. And always ensure that you're warmed up but not fatigued!

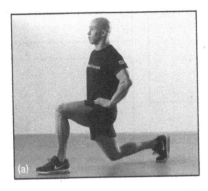

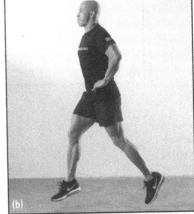

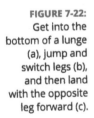

FIGURE 7-22:
Get into the bottom of a lunge (a), jump and switch legs (b), and then land with the opposite leg forward (c).

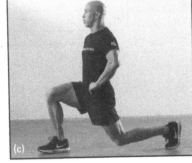

Photo by Jorge Alvarez, www.alvarezphoto.com

Practicing the Kneeling Transitions

Kneeling transitions are basically lunging movements that are performed from the ground up. Improving these transitions helps you develop useful postural habits and control your weight shifting where it counts most.

Long kneeling transitions

The long kneeling transition uses a relatively big step to transition between a double-kneeling and standing position. Just like with regular lunges, keep your midsection tight and your torso vertical.

1. Get into a double-kneeling position, as shown in Figure 7-23a.

2. Shift your weight onto your right hip and step forward with your left leg while bringing your arms to the T position. Place your left foot far enough in front of your trailing knee so that 90 degree angles are formed at the ankles, knees, and hips, as shown in Figure 7-23b.

3. Shift your weight onto your left leg and stand with your arms at the T position, as shown in Figure 7-23c.

4. Reverse the movement to get back to the double-kneeling position. Then switch sides.

As with all these kneeling transitions, you can do them with different arm positions. Holding the arms to the front makes the exercise easier. Using the streamline position makes the exercise harder.

Short kneeling transitions

This movement uses a squat-like position to transition between kneeling and standing positions. It's a bit harder than the long kneeling transition, so it's best to first get the hang of that exercise before trying this one.

1. Get into a double-kneeling position, as shown in Figure 7-24a.

2. Place your left foot flat on the ground next to your right knee, as shown in Figure 7-24b. You need to push your hips back to get your foot flat on the ground. Lift your chest and perform a big arm swing to place your hands behind your head.

3. Stand up straight with your feet hip-width apart and your toes pointing straight ahead, as shown in Figure 7-24c.

4. Reverse the movement to get back to an extended double-kneeling position, and then switch sides.

As you transition from a double-kneeling position to a short kneeling position, you need to push your hips back to get your forward foot flat on the ground. Once your heel is on the ground, lift your chest and perform an arm swing to get your arms into position. Here again, you can use different arm positions to vary the focus and difficulty.

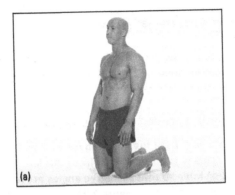
(a)

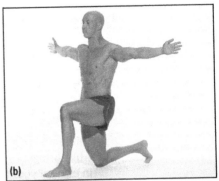
(b)

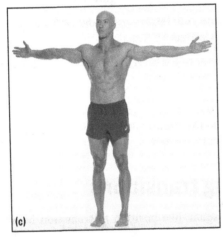
(c)

FIGURE 7-23:
Be sure to keep your midsection tight and your torso vertical.

Photo by Jorge Alvarez, www.alvarezphoto.com

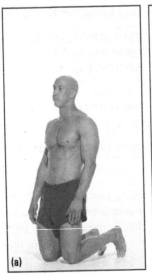
(a)

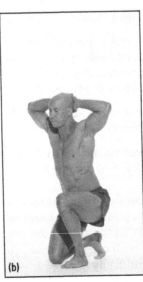
(b)

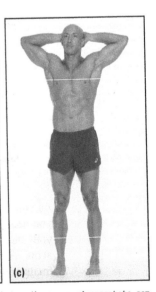
(c)

FIGURE 7-24:
The extended double-kneeling exercise.

Photo by Jorge Alvarez, www.alvarezphoto.com

Side kneeling transitions

This transition is slightly more complex, but it is well worth the effort of learning. With this movement, you'll develop the hip mobility and coordination needed for better lateral (side-to-side) movement.

1. Get into a double-kneeling position, as shown in Figure 7-25a.

2. Shift your weight onto your right hip and extend your left leg to the left side, as shown in Figure 7-25b. The toes of your left foot should face straight ahead.

3. Push your hips back and place your hands on the ground in front of your right knee, as shown in Figure 7-25c.

4. Shift your weight onto your left leg by straightening your right leg and bending your left leg until you're in the position shown in Figure 7-25d.

5. Stand up straight, as shown in Figure 7-25e, by straightening your left leg and dragging your right foot to your left foot.

After standing up, reverse the movement to get back to a double-kneeling position. In the beginning, it'll be easier for you to practice just one side at a time. Once you get more proficient with this exercise, you can start alternating sides after every rep.

TIP

If you want detailed video tutorials for this exercise and many others, go to the Instagram page *Mark_Lauren_Bodyweight*. You'll find a link in the bio that gives you access to all the free videos in the subscription app, *Mark Lauren On Demand*.

Bottom squats

The bottom squat is similar to the squat to lunge exercise except that you're starting from a double-kneeling position instead of a standing position. This exercise helps you gain greater control of your hips, which are literally at the center of everything you do!

1. Start in a double-kneeling position, as shown in Figure 7-26a.

2. Step forward with your left leg into a single kneeling position, as shown in Figure 7-26b. Raise your arms straight in front and push your hips back slightly.

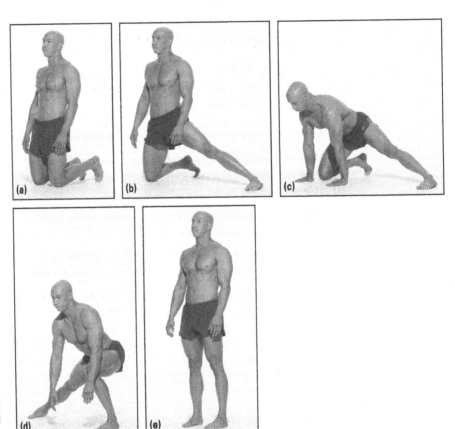

FIGURE 7-25: This exercise helps build hip mobility and lateral coordination.

Photo by Jorge Alvarez, www.alvarezphoto.com

3. Shift your weight onto your left leg. While keeping your hips low and your chest up, climb into the bottom of a squat, as shown in Figure 7-26c.

4. Reverse the movement to get back to a double-kneeling position and then switch sides.

As you transition from a single kneeling position to a squat, only the trailing leg should move. Work on keeping all the other parts of your body still. The elevation of your hips should not change.

Cossack squats

This incredible exercise improves your ability to move laterally while strengthening and lengthening all the muscles of your legs and hips. It's a tough one, but don't worry. You can also try an easier variation that allows you to build up to this.

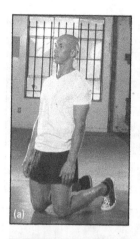
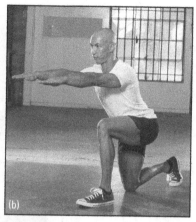
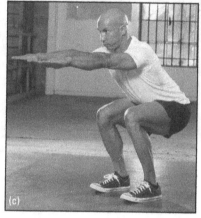

FIGURE 7-26:
Work on keeping all the other parts of your body still during this movement.

Photo by Jorge Alvarez, www.alvarezphoto.com

1. Start in a double-kneeling position, as shown in Figure 7-27a.

2. Step forward with your right leg and get into a long single kneeling position with your arms raised to the front, as shown in Figure 7-27b.

3. Rotate to the left and get into a side lunging position, as shown in Figure 7-27c.

4. Let your hips sink down as far as possible while keeping your right foot flat on the floor. Lift your chest, and fully straighten your left leg while turning the toes and knee of your left leg straight up toward the sky, as shown in Figure 7-27d. Reverse the movement to get back to a double-kneeling position. Then switch sides.

If Step 4 is too difficult, stop at Step 3 and reverse the movement to get back to a double-kneeling position before switching sides.

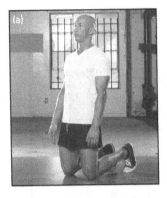
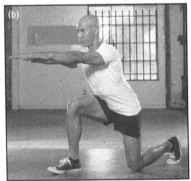
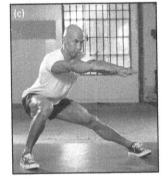
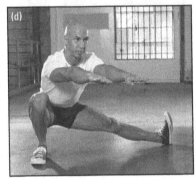

FIGURE 7-27:
This exercise
strengthens all
the muscles
of your legs
and hips.

Photo by Jorge Alvarez, www.alvarezphoto.com

Strengthening with Step-Ups

Step-ups are relatively simple exercises that have a great carry over to improved real life performance, because they involve simultaneous hip flexion and hip extension, as well as control weight shifting (balance). They're similar to lunging movements in this regard, except that with step-ups, only the foot of the extended hip is in contact with the ground. Lunges and step-ups complement each other well.

Stork stances

This is the basis and starting point for all step-up movements. Regardless of your level of advancement, it's a good idea to regularly revisit this simple movement.

1. **Stand with your feet hip-width apart and toes pointing straight ahead, as shown in Figure 7-28a. Place your arms in the T position.**

2. **Lift your left knee as high as possible while standing up as straight as possible, as shown in Figure 7-28b.**

3. Keep your supporting leg straight. Tighten your abdominals and lift your chest slightly. Switch sides after each rep.

Make yourself as tall as possible in the standing positions. Fully extend through your hips, lift your chest, and tighten your abs as if you might get punched in the gut at any moment. Get your knees up as high as you can while fully extending through the supporting leg so that you're as straight as humanly possible. You should feel an awesome squeeze in your glute. Also, pull the toes of the raised foot up, as if you're marching in place.

FIGURE 7-28:
Stand with your arms in a T-arm position (a) and then lift your left knee as high as possible (b).

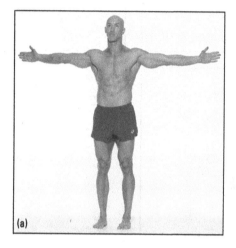 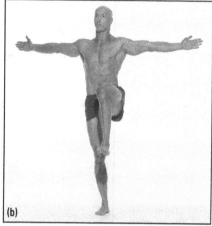

Photo by Jorge Alvarez, www.alvarezphoto.com

Gate swings

This exercise builds on the stork stance with external hip rotation at the top of the movement, which is often needed when we step over objects.

1. Stand with your arms in a T-arm position, as shown in Figure 7-29a.

2. While keeping your supporting leg and upper body straight, lift your left knee as high as possible, as shown in Figure 7-29b.

3. From the top position, rotate your left knee to the outside, as shown in Figure 7-29c, while pulling your right shoulder blade back to prevent movement through your upper body. Bring your left knee back to the center and then lower your leg to complete one rep.

Just like with the stork stance, focus on keeping your body as straight as possible. Get your knee up as high as you can while keeping your torso straight.

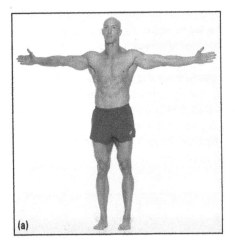
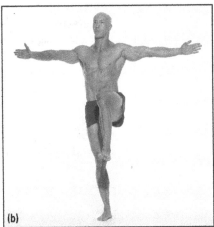

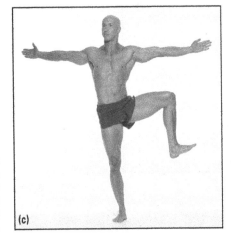

Photo by Jorge Alvarez, www.alvarezphoto.com

FIGURE 7-29: This exercise builds on the stork stance with an external hip rotation.

Cross steps

This exercise also builds on the stork stance by adding a step across your body's center line, which we commonly do when changing direction. An example of this is turning left by stepping across your body's center line with your right foot while walking.

REMEMBER

It's not just about burning calories and building muscle. You can also build useful athletic ability that improves performance and prevents injury. You can accomplish that by focusing your limited time and energy on the athletic skills most commonly used. By improving the basic building blocks of athletic ability, you'll get the most for the least.

1. Stand with your arms in the T position, as shown in Figure 7-30a.

2. Get into a good stork stance position by lifting your left leg as high as possible while keeping your torso up right, as shown in Figure 7-30b.

3. Step across your right foot with your left foot, as shown in Figure 7-30b. As you step across the supporting right foot with the left foot, draw your left shoulder blade back. See Figure 7-30c.

4. In the bottom position, position your elevated foot as if it's about to support the weight of your body. Lift your left knee to get back to stork stance and then return to the starting position.

This exercise often alleviates discomfort in the lower back area, because it involves side to side tilting of the pelvis, which is overlooked in most exercise programs. As you perform this movement, pay attention to how your pelvis is moving. The left side of your pelvis should rise slightly as you lift your left leg, and it should fall as you lower your left leg to step across your right foot.

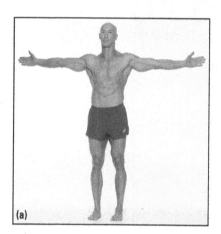

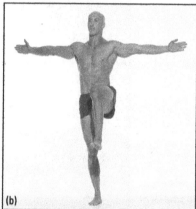

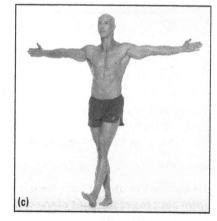

FIGURE 7-30: The cross step exercise builds on the stork stance by adding a step across your body's center line.

Photo by Jorge Alvarez, www.alvarezphoto.com

High-knee marches

This movement improves posture, hip mobility, and coordination.

1. **March in place. Stand up straight, keep your feet parallel, and find a steady pace.**

2. **Bring your knees up high, as shown in Figure 7-31, and use a strong arm swing while keeping your elbows bent at 90 degrees.**

With each step, fully extend through the supporting leg while lifting your chest slightly and keeping your abs tensed. Get your knees up and swing your arms with your elbows bent at 90 degrees. This basic movement pattern has a lot of useful carry over to real-life activities when it's done properly.

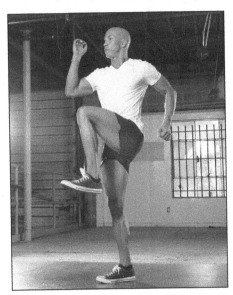

FIGURE 7-31:
Marching in place with good posture.

Photo by Jorge Alvarez, www.alvarezphoto.com

High-knee runs

The difference between the high-knee march and high-knee run is that when you're marching, one foot is always in contact with the floor. When you're running, the planted foot comes up as the raised foot comes down. Of course, that's actually also one of the main differences between regular walking and running. Running has a "flight phase."

1. **Fully extend through the leg that's in contact with the floor, while thrusting the opposite arm back to get the knee of the opposite leg as high as you can, as shown in Figure 7-32.**

2. **Keep your midsection tight and lean forward slightly. Focus more on high knees and less on speed. As your raised knee comes down, your other knee should already be coming up.**

Focus on your posture by lifting your chest slightly while keeping your midsection tight. Make yourself straight, with a slight forward lean. Energetically swing your arms and get your knees up.

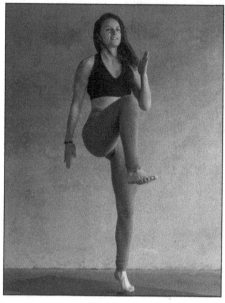

FIGURE 7-32:
Running in place with high knees and a strong arm swing.

Photo courtesy of Emka Photography

High-knee skips

You're skipping in place. If you're one of those few who already know how to do it, wonderful. But for those of us who don't, it can take practice.

1. **Begin by running in place, nice and easy. Keep your knees low for now.**

2. **After a few steps on each side, add one-second pauses to each step, so that you're briefly holding up each knee. Get the rhythm of that.**

3. **Next, add a small one-legged hop to each step, as shown in Figure 7-33. You should now be skipping in place!**

As you improve, you'll be able to get your knees up higher and use a stronger arm swing. If you can't get the high-knee skip down, use the high-knee run or high-knee march instead.

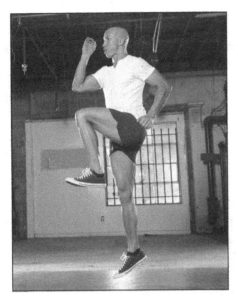

FIGURE 7-33:
Skipping in place
with high knees.

Photo by Jorge Alvarez, www.alvarezphoto.com

Chapter **8**

Pushing to Strengthen Your Chest, Shoulders, and Triceps

I n this chapter, you learn all about the exercises that you can do to develop your chest, shoulders, and triceps by way of pushing against force, be it your own body weight or other objects in your environment. The chapter starts by explaining how to maintain ideal alignment. Then it gets into the practical part — the actual exercises!

WARNING

It's always a good idea to check with your doctor before you begin an exercise regimen. Also, if any of the exercises in this chapter cause you pain, stop doing them. It's important to be able to recognize the difference between something that is hard and something this is painful. No exercise should cause pain. Always listen to your body.

Maintaining Ideal Alignment Under Stress

Aside from targeting the muscles of your chest, shoulders, and triceps, pushing movements with bodyweight exercises strengthen and stabilize your core about as well as core exercises themselves. And that's because in real life, when you need to overcome force by pushing something, like a door or even a car, your *anterior* core (the front of your core) has to be engaged in order to maintain the alignment needed for an effective transfer of energy.

When you're performing these exercises, don't just think about the joints that are moving, also pay attention to the rest of your body to ensure that you remain as straight as possible through all the parts that should not be moving.

Practicing the Perpendicular Pushing Exercises

These are pushing movements with your arms perpendicular to your torso, such as push-ups. The focus with this arm position tends to be more on the chest and triceps and less on the shoulders.

TIP

For specific guidance on how to use these exercises in a routine, check out the 13-week program in Chapter 12. You can also find many more exercise programs for varying fitness levels, as well as video tutorials, via the marklauren.com website. Use promo code STRONG15 to save 15 percent on annual memberships.

Classic push-ups

The key to doing push-ups properly is getting a full range of motion while maintaining a straight body position from head to heels.

1. Lie down on your stomach, feet together, with your hands directly below your shoulders, as shown in Figure 8-1a.

2. Push yourself up off the ground until your arms are fully extended and your shoulders are slightly protracted, so that you feel your shoulder blades pulling away from each other, as shown in Figure 8-1b.

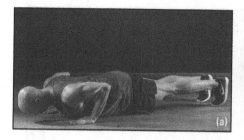
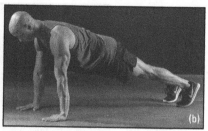

Photo by Jorge Alvarez, www.alvarezphoto.com

FIGURE 8-1:
Lie down on your stomach (a) and then push yourself all the way up (b).

Throughout the entire movement, your body should be in a straight line. From your heels to your neck, nothing should be bent. Be especially certain not to let your pelvis drop toward the ground, or let your butt stick up in the air at all. Weak form means a weak core. Keep your midsection tight!

You can adjust the difficulty of this exercise by using a sturdy surface to elevate your hands or feet. By elevating your hands, as shown in Figure 8-2, you'll make the exercise easier. You can also do push-ups with your knees on the ground. By elevating your feet, as shown in Figure 8-3, you'll make the exercise harder.

TIP

The best way to overcome difficult exercises is by focusing on a controlled negative. That means controlling the way down over about a three-five second count. In the case of difficult pushing exercises, you simply cheat yourself up to the top position using a worm-type movement, getting into good alignment, and then doing your best to control and decelerate the descent. Worm yourself back up to the top and repeat.

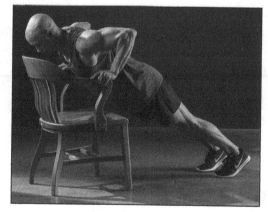

FIGURE 8-2:
Elevate your hands to make push-ups easier.

Photo by Jorge Alvarez, www.alvarezphoto.com

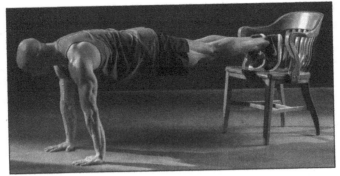

FIGURE 8-3:
Elevate your
feet to make
push-ups harder.

Photo by Jorge Alvarez, www.alvarezphoto.com

Staggered push-ups

This is a push-up variation with your hands positioned asymmetrically, which makes it harder to keep your body in a straight line. Someone standing directly above you should see a straight line from your head to your heels.

1. **This is performed just like a classic push-up except one hand is slightly forward of the normal position and the other hand is slightly back, as shown in Figure 8-4a.**

2. **Lower yourself fully to the ground, as shown in Figure 8-4b, and then push yourself back up.**

Switch hand positions every other set. This is a great exercise for attacking your muscles with varying stimulus.

FIGURE 8-4:
The starting
position (a) and
ending position
(b) for staggered
push-ups.

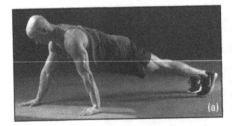 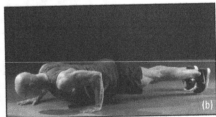

Photo by Jorge Alvarez, www.alvarezphoto.com

Archer push-ups

These push-ups resemble an archer drawing a bow, hence the name archer push-ups. This is one of the more difficult push-up variations, so I recommend being able to do regular push-ups with your feet elevated to knee height before attempting these.

1. Get into push-up position with your feet hip-width apart and your hands wider than shoulder-width apart, as shown in Figure 8-5a. Position your hands so that your fingers are pointing to the sides.

2. While keeping your body straight, lower yourself to your right hand, as shown in Figure 8-5b, and then return to the starting position.

3. Lower yourself to your left side, as shown in Figure 8-5c, to complete the rep.

You can make this exercise easier by resting your knees on the ground. A good way to develop strength with difficult exercises is to do a lot of low rep sets with plenty of rest. Avoid making yourself tired to the point that you can no longer maintain proper form.

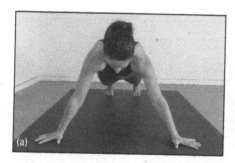

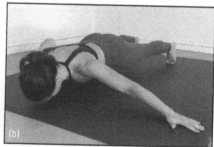

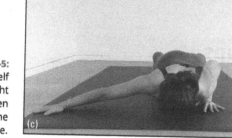

FIGURE 8-5: Lower yourself fully to the right side and then fully to the left side.

Photo courtesy of Lea Badenhoop

Contra presses

These are excellent one-arm push-up variations that give you a lot of options for varying difficulty. After the description for the standard variation, you'll find ways to make the movement easier.

1. Lie down on your stomach in the starting position of a push-up and grab the inside of your left thigh with your left hand, as shown in Figure 8-6a.

2. While maintaining a straight line from your head to your right heel, push yourself off the ground, as shown in Figure 8-6b.

3. Lower yourself fully to complete the rep.

There are several ways to make this exercise easier:

>> You can place the knee of your extended leg on the ground.

>> You can let go of the inside of your thigh and push yourself up with both arms.

>> You can use both arms to push yourself up and keep both knees on the ground.

FIGURE 8-6:
The contra
press has many
variations.

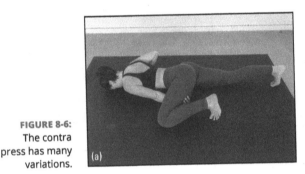
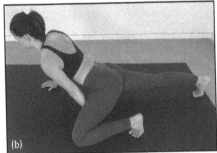

Photo courtesy of Lea Badenhoop

Tripod push-ups

This exercise is similar to one-arm push-ups in that there are only three points of contact with the ground, which creates the need to resist and control rotation. With one-arm push-ups, you have one hand and both feet in contact with the ground. With tripod push-ups, both hands and one foot are in contact with the ground. The advantage of this variation is that it's easier to scale the difficulty of tripod push-ups.

1. Get into a push-up position with your hands and feet shoulder-width apart. Tense your glutes and tighten your midsection. Raise your left leg off the floor and keep the knee and toes of the elevated leg pointing straight down, as shown in Figure 8-7a.

2. **Lower yourself to the floor while keeping your body straight, as shown in Figure 8-7b. Drive yourself back up.**

Do two reps with the left leg elevated, and then do two reps with the right leg elevated.

This exercise gets harder the wider your feet are apart, and it likewise gets easier with your feet closer together. If this exercise is too difficult, try working yourself back up to the starting position and focus on controlling the way down with a straight body position.

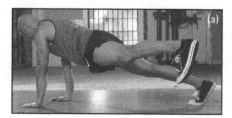 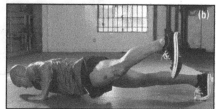

Photo by Jorge Alvarez, www.alvarezphoto.com

Dips

Dips are an incredible exercise for developing your lower chest, the front of your shoulders, and your triceps.

1. **Find any two stable surfaces that are, or can be positioned, a couple of feet apart. The two surfaces should be equal in height and at least waist high.**

2. **Place a palm on each surface, lock your arms out straight to your sides, bend your knees, and suspend your body between the surfaces, as shown in Figure 8-8a.**

3. **Lower yourself as far as possible, your knees suspended in the air above the ground, as shown in Figure 8-8b, and then push yourself back up.**

You can assist yourself by using your legs to push off the ground. And just like with push-up variations, you can cheat yourself to the top and do your best to control the way down.

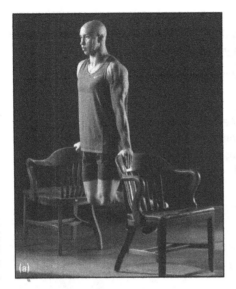
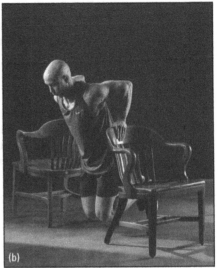

FIGURE 8-8:
The starting position (a) and ending position (b) for dips.

Seated dips

This variation of dips is significantly easier than regular dips while working the same muscles. Aside from being easier, this variation will give you more of a stretch through the front of your shoulders, which makes it a nice stretching movement after long periods of typing or playing on your phone.

1. Find a horizontal surface between knee and waist-level. The lower the surface is, the more difficult this exercise gets, but it can't be below knee level. A table, chair, futon, or couch armrest will all do the trick.

2. With your back to the surface, place your palms on the edge of the surface behind you, your knuckles pointing forward, as shown in Figure 8-9a.

3. Lower your body straight down bending only at the elbows and shoulders, until your upper arms are parallel to the floor, as shown in Figure 8-9b, or until you get a gentle stretch in your shoulders. Push yourself back up until your arms are straight again.

You can make the exercise slightly more difficult by straightening your legs, as shown in Figure 8-9c. To make the movement still more difficult, elevate your feet on something about knee height, such as a chair.

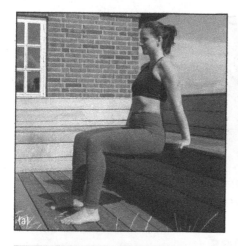
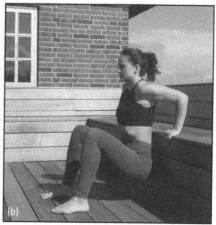
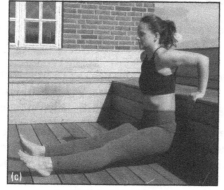

FIGURE 8-9:
In the ending
position,
the upper arms
are parallel to
the ground.

Photo courtesy of Lea Badenhoop

Bouncing push-ups

This exercise builds explosive power. It's the same as a classic push-up, but you're pushing yourself up so hard and fast that your hands come up off the ground at the top of the movement when your arms are straight (see Figure 8-10). When you return to Earth, don't let your hands crash back down on the floor. Instead, land with soft hands, wrists, and elbows to absorb the force, then tighten your arms and shoulders for the next explosive repetition.

You can do this exercise from your knees to make it easier. You can also elevate your hands on a sturdy hip-high surface such as a countertop.

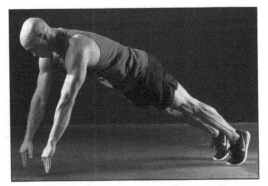

FIGURE 8-10:
An explosive
push-up
variation.

Semi-planches

Make sure you're properly warmed-up before doing this exercise. This push-up variation places a lot of emphasis on the front of your shoulders.

1. Lie flat on your stomach with your toes pointed straight back on the ground. Place your hands, palms down, near your lower ribs so that your fingers are pointing back toward your toes, as shown in Figure 8-11a.

2. Push yourself up until your arms are straight, as shown in Figure 8-11b. Flex your glutes and draw your naval in toward your spine to make your back perfectly straight. Lower yourself in a controlled manner.

To make this exercise harder, start with your hands closer to your waist. A small change in the position of your hands will make a big difference in difficulty.

FIGURE 8-11:
The semi-planche
starting (a) and
ending (b)
position.

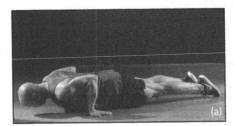
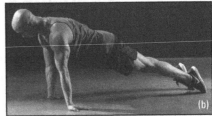

One-arm push-ups

This is a really tough exercise to do perfectly, because it requires a tremendous amount of core strength to maintain a straight body position. Probably for that reason, it's not a natural progression from mastering a lot of other types of push-ups.

I've seen plenty of people knock out 80 perfect non-stop push-ups, and yet they didn't have the strength and coordination to do a single proper one-arm push-up. With that said, tripod push-ups and the contra press have a much better carry-over to one-arm push-ups.

1. **Get into push-up position with your feet slightly wider than shoulder-width apart and your hands close together so that your thumbs can touch. Now place your right hand on your lower back, as shown in Figure 8-12a.**

2. **Tighten your midsection and lower yourself to the ground while keeping your hips and shoulders level (see Figure 8-12b).**

3. **To get back to the starting position, push yourself back up with a straight and level body position (very hard), or worm yourself back up (easier).**

To make this exercise much easier, place your hands on a sturdy countertop. As you get stronger, place your hands on progressively lower surfaces, such as the chair shown in Figure 8-12c. If you use a chair, back it against a wall so that it doesn't slide around.

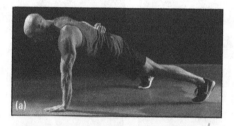
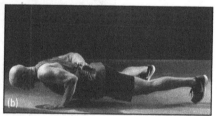
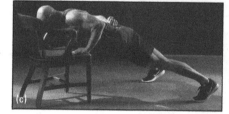

FIGURE 8-12:
The one-arm push-up requires a tremendous amount of strength.

Photo by Jorge Alvarez, www.alvarezphoto.com

Trying the Inline Pushing Exercises

For these pushing exercises your hands will be in line with your torso (think handstand). This places more of an emphasis on your shoulders, triceps, and trapezius, and less on your chest.

Military presses

This is a classic that I did a lot of as a Special Operations trainee in the U.S. Air Force.

1. Stand with your heels together and place your hands in front of your feet, as shown in Figure 8-13a.

2. Count five hand lengths away from your feet and place your hands on the ground slightly wider than shoulder-width apart, as shown in Figure 8-13b. Push your chest down toward your feet and try to straighten your legs.

3. Keeping everything but your arms in a fixed position, your back straight and your butt in the air, bend your arms at the elbow until the top of your head almost touches the ground between your hands, as shown in Figure 8-13c. Then push yourself back up to the starting position.

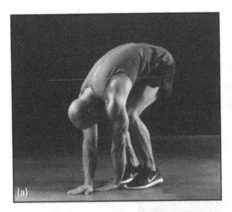
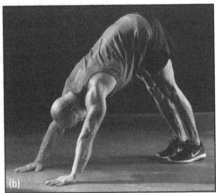
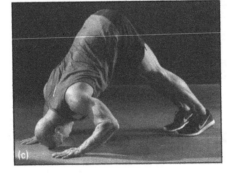

FIGURE 8-13: The military press stretches your hamstrings while working your shoulders and triceps.

Photo by Jorge Alvarez, www.alvarezphoto.com

As you bend your arms to lower and raise yourself, point your elbows toward your feet slightly. Your elbows shouldn't flare out completely and they shouldn't be completely tucked. They should be somewhere in the middle.

If you're doing this exercise correctly, you should feel a stretch in your hamstrings unless you're very flexible. Do your best to keep your legs and back straight.

TIP

For an easier variation, place your hands on an elevated surface, as shown in Figure 8-14. Placing your feet on an elevated surface, such as in Figure 8-15, will make this exercise more difficult.

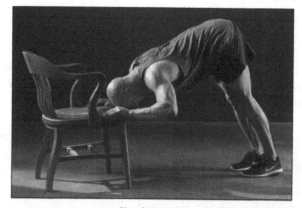

FIGURE 8-14: Elevate your hands to make the exercise easier.

Photo by Jorge Alvarez, www.alvarezphoto.com

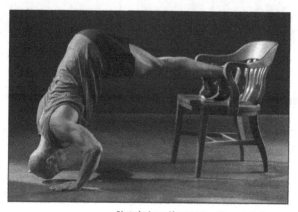

FIGURE 8-15: Elevate your feet to make the exercise harder.

Photo by Jorge Alvarez, www.alvarezphoto.com

Dive bombers

This exercise is great for developing both strength and flexibility.

1. Get into the starting position of a push-up with your feet hip-width apart and your hands shoulder-width apart.

2. Push your hips up into the air and push your chest down toward your feet, as shown in Figure 8-16a. Let your heels sink to the ground. You should feel a stretch in your hamstrings.

3. Lower your hips straight to the ground and lift your chest, as shown in Figure 8-16b.

   Take a moment to let yourself sink into position while looking straight ahead. Pull your shoulders back and open your chest.

Take the time to get a good stretch in each end position. At the top, push your chest down toward your feet and straighten your legs. Let your heels sink down. At the bottom, pull your shoulders back.

FIGURE 8-16:
The dive bomber
starting (a) and
ending (b)
position.

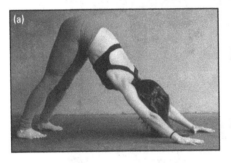 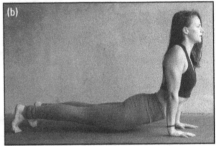

Photo courtesy of Lea Badenhoop

DF glides

This exercise combines the dive bomber and classic push-up to evenly develop your chest, shoulders, and triceps.

1. Get to the bottom position of a push-up with your feet hip-width apart and your wrists directly under your shoulders, as shown in Figure 8-17a.

2. Push yourself up as you would for a regular push-up, as shown in Figure 8-17b.

3. Push your hips up into the air while pushing your chest down toward your feet, as shown in Figure 8-17c. Let your heels sink down toward the floor. You should feel a good stretch in the back of your legs.

4. **Reverse the movement and lower yourself directly to the bottom of a push-up to complete the repetition.**

Think of this exercise as a push-up where you push your hips up into the air to get a good stretch after every rep. To make this exercise easier, worm yourself up to the starting position of a push-up, and then get your hips up into the air. Focus on a controlled descent with a long, straight body position at the end.

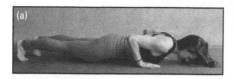
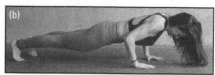
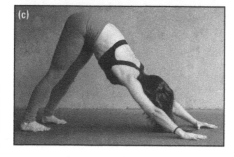

FIGURE 8-17:
This exercise combines the dive bomber and classic push-up.

Photo courtesy of Lea Badenhoop

Bear crawls

This is a fun and effective exercise that works your shoulders, upper back, arms, core, hips, and legs. It's a total body exercise.

Simply place your hands on the ground a few feet in front of your toes and start crawling on your hands and feet (see Figure 8-18). Have some fun. This is a great exercise to do at the end of your workout.

There are several variations to this exercise:

>> **Contralateral:** Move your left hand and right foot at the same time and then your right hand and left foot.

>> **Ipsilateral:** Move your left hand and left foot at the same time, and then your right hand and right foot.

You can do both variations of this exercise going forward and backward. Enjoy!

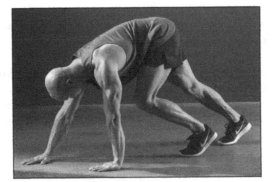

FIGURE 8-18:
The bear
crawl — RAHH!!

Photo by Jorge Alvarez, www.alvarezphoto.com

Chapter **9**

Pulling Exercises to Strengthen Your Back, Biceps, and Forearms

I f you want a strong, healthy body that is fully balanced and resistant to high levels of stress, you'll need to do pulling exercises to develop your lats, upper back, biceps, and forearms. Not only will you be able to lift yourself and external objects with greater security, your posture will be more stable with strong lats, which connect everything from your arms and shoulder blades to your pelvis.

Doing pulling movements does require a bit of equipment. However, with a bit of creativity, you can almost always find a safe way to do pulling exercises just about anywhere. The following sections give you some tips.

WARNING

It's always a good idea to check with your doctor before you begin an exercise regimen. Also, if any of the exercises in this chapter cause you pain, stop doing them. It's important to be able to recognize the difference between something that is hard and something this is painful. No exercise should cause pain. Always listen to your body.

Finding Tools for Pulling Exercises

To do these exercises you need to find sturdy objects that can support your weight, such as a door, pole, railing, or desk. Although you certainly don't need to purchase anything, you can go to your local sporting goods store or Amazon.com to buy an inexpensive pull-up bar that hooks into a doorway, along with suspension straps that you can fasten to a doorway or the pull-up bar itself. You'll see some of these objects in the images in this chapter. Some playgrounds and parks also have rudimentary exercise bars and stations along their walkways that you can use when weather permits. Get creative!

TIP

If you want detailed video tutorials for many of these exercises, go to the Instagram page *Mark_Lauren_Bodyweight.* You'll find a link in the bio that gives you access to all the free videos in the subscription app, *Mark Lauren On Demand.*

Practicing Perpendicular Pulling Exercises

Perpendicular pulling exercises are pulling movements in which your arms are perpendicular to your torso. These movements are particularly good for your upper back. They are also easier than inline pulling exercises, where your arms are in line with your torso, as is the case with pull-ups. Perpendicular pulling exercises are therefore a useful stepping stone to inline pulling exercises.

The following sections go through several different perpendicular pulling exercises. Find the ones that work best for you. Remember that they should feel difficult but be not painful.

Let-me-ins

Let-me-ins are the easiest pulling movements and a great starting place for beginners. With that said, you can adjust the difficulty of these movements to allow for gradual progression to high levels.

1. **Find a sturdy door and loop a mid-sized towel over and under the handle, as shown in Figure 9-1.**

   You can also loop a towel around a sturdy pole or railing at about waist height, or you can even just grab the railing or pole instead of using a towel.

2. **Firmly grip one end of the towel in each hand. Place your feet 8-12 inches in front of your hands.**

   Ensure you have good traction and lower your hips until your knees are bent about 90 degrees and your arms are straight, as shown in Figure 9-2. Keep your knees bent at the same angle throughout the exercise.

3. **Next, pull your chest to your hands and squeeze your shoulder blades together, while keeping your midsection drawn in and your chest slightly elevated, as shown in Figure 9-3.**

   Pay attention to your posture and take a brief second to ensure you're in a good position with a neutral spine and your shoulders fully retracted. You can also pull the towel apart at this end position as if you're ripping a shirt open to show the Superman S on your chest.

4. **Return to the starting position by straightening your arms.**

   Before beginning the next rep, ensure you're positioned properly, as described in Step 2.

FIGURE 9-1: Find a sturdy door handle to anchor a hand towel for let-me-ins.

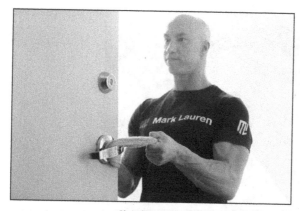

Photo by Jorge Alvarez, www.alvarezphoto.com

TIP

You can do let-me-ins using just one arm at a time, as shown in Figure 9-4. This version is obviously much harder, and it can be especially challenging for your grip. In these images, I'm using a towel wrapped around a swing, which works well, but you can do one-arm let-me-ins using a door, pole, or railing as well.

TIP

Moving your feet further forward will make this exercise harder. Moving them back some will make it easier. You need to be sure to have good traction with the floor, so it helps to wear shoes.

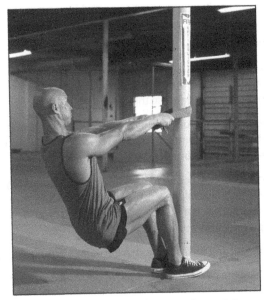

FIGURE 9-2:
Position your feet just in front of your hands, and lean back with your knees and hips bent.

Photo by Jorge Alvarez, www.alvarezphoto.com

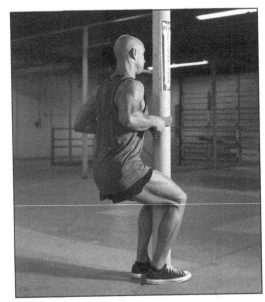

FIGURE 9-3:
At the top, ensure you have good posture by lifting your chest, flexing your abs, and pulling your shoulders back.

Photo by Jorge Alvarez, www.alvarezphoto.com

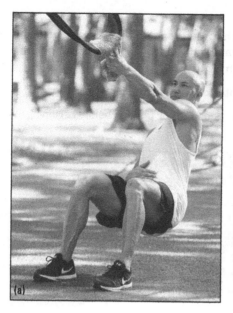
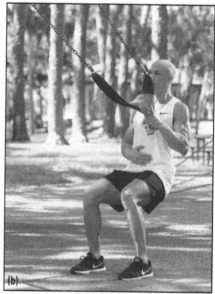

Photo by Jorge Alvarez, www.alvarezphoto.com

FIGURE 9-4: With the one-armed version, keep yourself straight and symmetrical, just like with regular let-me-ins.

WARNING

As you can see in Figure 9-4, there's plenty of room for creativity in terms of finding a way to do pulling exercises, so feel free to improvise. Just be sure that you're using things sturdy enough to support your weight, and make sure you have good traction, so your feet don't slide. Wearing shoes is recommended.

Let-me-ups

Once you're able to do two-arm let-me-ins with relative ease, you're ready to start working with let-me-ups. Similar to let-me-ins, let-me-ups are a pulling movement where your arms are perpendicular to your body. However, with let-me-ups, your body is horizontal instead of vertical. This exercise also has plenty of variations that allow you to scale the difficulty for long-term progression.

1. **Lie under a sturdy table that's about waist height. Reach up and grab the edges of the table with your hands about shoulder width apart, as shown in Figure 9-5a.**

   If the table is short, or you're tall, try taking a wide enough grip so that your back isn't touching the ground. Your legs should be bent at 90 degrees. This makes the exercise significantly easier than having your legs straight. It's also a great way to strengthen your glutes.

2. **Lift your chest up between your hands, squeezing your shoulder blades together, while maintaining a straight body position from your head to knees, as shown in Figure 9-5b.**

3. **Lower yourself until your arms are straight and repeat.**

   Be sure to reset to a good starting position before beginning the next rep.

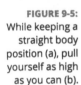

FIGURE 9-5:
While keeping a straight body position (a), pull yourself as high as you can (b).

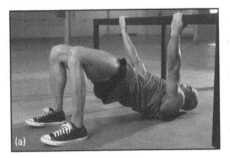 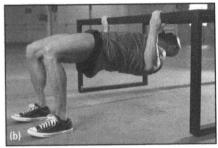

Photo by Jorge Alvarez, www.alvarezphoto.com

REMEMBER

All these movements should strengthen your muscles while ingraining useful postural habits, which allow you to stay long and straight while force is being applied from different angles. To make yourself straight, slightly lift your chest while tightening your abs and glutes.

TIP

Try using different hand positions to spice up your training. The added variety helps prevent plateaus while keeping things interesting and making you a more well-rounded athlete. The difficulty of these hand positions varies from person to person, so feel free to experiment.

Figure 9-5 and shows an underhand grip that places slightly more emphasis on the biceps. Figure 9-6 shows a neutral grip where the palms face each other, which distributes the work load more evenly between the arms and entire back. In Figure 9-7 an overhand grip is shown that puts more emphasis on your upper back, especially when a wide grip is used. Lastly, in Figure 9-8, you have an alternating grip, which is a good option if you find that your grip is a weak link.

TIP

You can make all of these variations more difficult by elevating your feet on something about knee height, such as a chair, stepladder, or stool, as shown in Figure 9-9. Be sure to make yourself straight from head to heels. Once you've mastered this variation, trying using just one leg to support yourself, as shown in Figure 9-10.

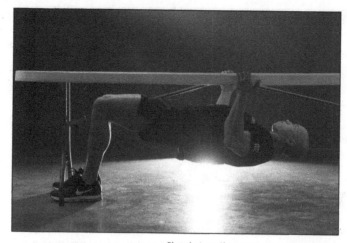

FIGURE 9-6:
Using a neutral grip more evenly distributes the work load.

Photo by Jorge Alvarez, www.alvarezphoto.com

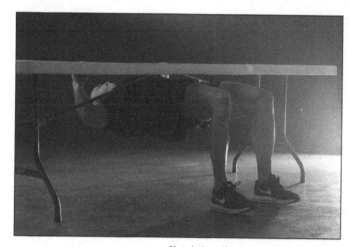

FIGURE 9-7:
You can use a variety of grips when doing let-me-ups on a desk or table.

Photo by Jorge Alvarez, www.alvarezphoto.com

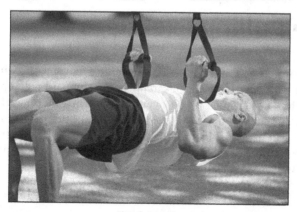

FIGURE 9-8:
Using an alternating grip makes it easier to hold on, especially when using a bar.

Photo by Jorge Alvarez, www.alvarezphoto.com

CHAPTER 9 Pulling Exercises to Strengthen Your Back, Biceps, and Forearms

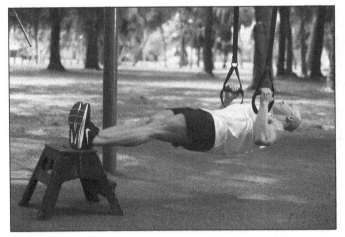

Photo by Jorge Alvarez, www.alvarezphoto.com

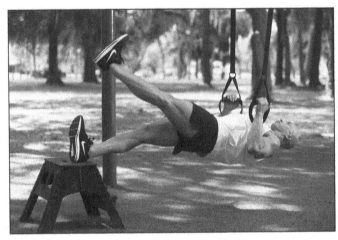

Photo by Jorge Alvarez, www.alvarezphoto.com

Trying Inline Pulling Exercises

The exercises covered in this section are pulling movements, whereby your arms are in line with your torso. One example is the standard pull-up. Although pull-ups and chin-ups may be beyond your abilities at this time, there are ways to adjust the difficulty of these exercises so that you can safely and effectively train your back and arms using these pulling movements. However, before you try these inline pulling exercises, first get comfortable with the perpendicular pulling movements covered earlier in this chapter.

Pull-ups

Pull-ups are a classic body-weight exercise that just about everyone is familiar with. While they are one of the more difficult exercises in this book, there are variations useful to everyone who has the strength to hang from a bar. Let's get started with the standard variation and then regress from there.

1. **Grab onto an overhead bar with your palms facing forward.**

   Your hands should be slightly wider than shoulder-width apart. Let yourself hang fully while making yourself as long as possible, as shown in Figure 9-11.

2. **While keeping yourself straight, pull yourself up as high as you can.**

   Ideally, you want to clear the bar with your chin while keeping your shoulders retracted, as shown in Figure 9-12.

3. **Lower yourself completely and get a good stretch at the bottom.**

   Getting into a long, straight position is the most important part of the pull-up, because it's this part of the movement that does the most for your strength and flexibility.

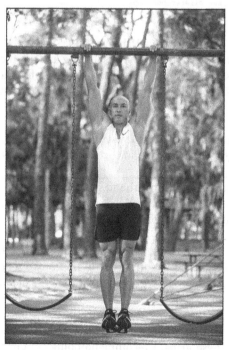

FIGURE 9-11: Make yourself as long as possible in the starting position of a pull-up.

Photo by Jorge Alvarez, www.alvarezphoto.com

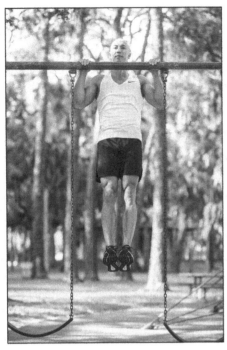

FIGURE 9-12: Pull yourself as high as you can while keeping a straight body position.

Photo by Jorge Alvarez, www.alvarezphoto.com

It's okay if you can't pull yourself all the way up. Quarter- and half-reps are totally acceptable. Just be sure to make yourself long and sat the end of each rep. If you can't pull yourself up at all, that's also okay. Simply practice short hangs while making yourself as straight as possible. This will do a lot to improve grip strength and shoulder health.

This is a difficult exercise that almost everyone struggles with. A great training strategy is using a high volume of very low-repetition sets or even just singles.

TIP

You can do this exercise with an underhand grip, as shown in Figure 9-13. This variation is known as chin-ups, which places more emphasis on the biceps. Most users find it easier than the overhand variation.

If grip strength is a problem for you, use an alternating grip with your palms facing in opposite directions, as shown in Figure 9-14. Do two repetitions at a time, and then switch hand positions. This gives you the benefits of both hand positions while making it easier to hold on.

You can further vary your training by using narrow, shoulder-width, or wide hand positions with any of these grips. I recommend doing so! Consistently applying small variations to your exercises, workout-to-workout, or even set-to-set, is a great way to prevent overtraining and plateaus.

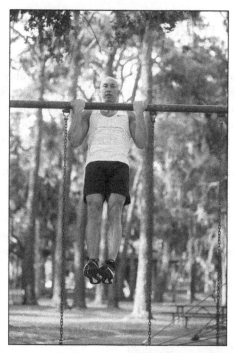

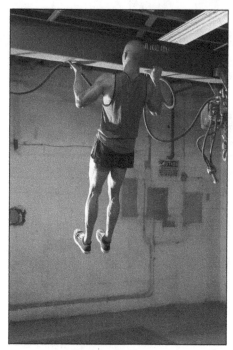

Assisted and negative pull-ups

You can make any of these variations easier using a variety of tools. In Figures 9-15 and 9-16, I've placed my foot in a suspension trainer to assist myself, but you could also use an exercise band or bands and place your foot or knee inside of them. The greater the tension of a band, the more it'll help you. Having a variety of bands allows you more options for adjusting the difficulty of this exercise. Amazon.com and your local sporting goods stores have a wide selection.

TIP

One of my favorite strength training techniques for pull-ups is using slow "negatives" where I "cheat" myself up to the top position by jumping or pushing off of something like a chair, and then lowering myself slowly unassisted over about a three to five-second count. Negative pull-ups can be combined with bands, if needed. Just be sure to not overdo it. This exercise variation can make you really sore! I use this variation at the end of my pulling sessions to get a few extra reps once I'm too tired for regular unassisted pull-ups. Don't forget that you can vary your hand positions and grips as well.

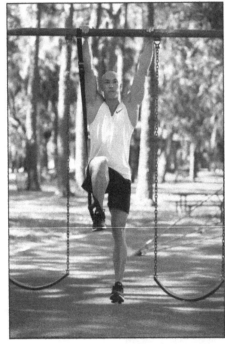

Photo by Jorge Alvarez, www.alvarezphoto.com

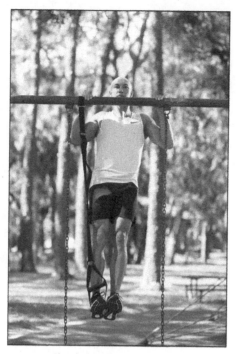

FIGURE 9-16:
Using controlled "negatives" is a great strength training tool. Cheat yourself up and control the way down! You can apply this to many exercises, including push-ups.

Photo by Jorge Alvarez, www.alvarezphoto.com

Chapter **10**

Exercises for Mobility

Both performance and injury resistance depend on getting into and maintaining ideal joint alignment. Your body depends on the correct alignment of its parts in order to tolerate stress, just like any other structure, such as bridges and buildings. The difference is that you're much more complex and constantly in motion. Thankfully, with the right movements and routines, learning to get into better alignment isn't complicated. It just takes consistent practice and persistence.

The exercises in this chapter are all built to help expand your mobility in everyday activities. Mobility is key to athletic health, so don't skip these practices! If you're starting this journey with limited mobility, be sure to check out Chapter 14 as well.

WARNING

It's always a good idea to check with your doctor before you begin an exercise regimen. Also, if any of the exercises in this chapter cause you pain, stop doing them. It's important to be able to recognize the difference between something that is hard and something this is painful. No exercise should cause pain. Always listen to your body.

Enjoying the Benefits of Proper Positioning

Mobility is a skill set that requires more than just flexibility, which can be described as the passive range of motion in joints. Mobility is about active positioning, which requires flexibility, coordination, and strength. Put very simply, mobility is the ability to "get there."

For mobility, the dominant qualities are flexibility and coordination. Stability is more dependent on strength, because it's your ability to maintain wanted positions, especially while force is acting against you. You could say that mobility is the ability to move while stability is the ability to not move. The interplay of mobility and stability allows you to move through space efficiently by getting you into ideal alignment and keeping you there.

Starting with the Spiderman Exercises

These movements start in a planking position with one leg forward so that the lead foot is next your hand, as shown in Figure 10-1. This position opens up your hips by lengthening the hip flexor of the rear leg and hamstring of the lead leg.

If you can't get your foot all the way forward next to your hand, just get it as close as you can. With regular practice, your range of motion will improve inch by inch. If you can get your leg all the way forward, make your entire body as long and straight as possible while keeping the knee of the lead leg pinned to your shoulder.

TIP

To access detailed video tutorials of these Mobility Exercises, go to the Instagram page *Mark_Lauren_Bodyweight*. You'll find a link in the bio that gives you access to all the free videos in the subscription app, *Mark Lauren On Demand*.

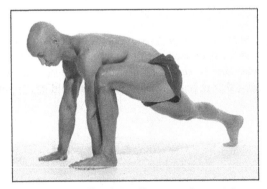

FIGURE 10-1:
Spiderman
starting position.

Photo by Jorge Alvarez, www.alvarezphoto.com

Hip swirls

The main purpose of this exercise is to get you into a better starting position for the Spiderman exercises. This is accomplished by having you make horizontal circles with your hips while in the starting position, which will create space by loosening up your hips.

1. **After getting into your best Spiderman starting position, begin by rocking your entire body forward, as shown in Figure 10-2.**

2. **From this position, move your hips and shoulders as a single unit in a clockwise motion, so that you're making horizontal circles.**

   After a few repetitions reverse directions and make counterclockwise circles. See Figure 10-3.

Start with small circles that get progressively bigger with each repetition. Once you reverse directions, start with small circles again that gradually increase in size. This exercise can be a bit awkward at first, so be patient. You'll soon develop the mobility and coordination needed to move more easily.

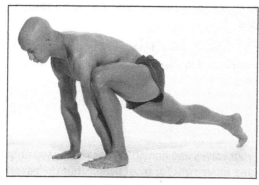

FIGURE 10-2: Make horizontal circles with your entire body.

Photo by Jorge Alvarez, www.alvarezphoto.com

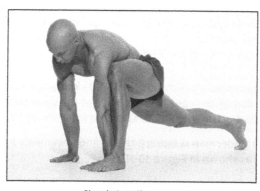

FIGURE 10-3: Keep your hips low and your forward knee pinned to your shoulder.

Photo by Jorge Alvarez, www.alvarezphoto.com

Getting your foot up next to your hand for the Spiderman starting position is much easier if you first shift your weight laterally. For example, to move your left leg forward, first shift your hips to the right. Then move the left leg forward. That lateral weight shift creates space for you to move your leg forward.

Arm circles

This exercise improves spinal rotation and overall shoulder mobility by challenging you to draw a giant circle with the arm next to your lead leg. In the beginning, you probably won't be able to position perfectly and that's to be expected. The progress from these exercises comes mainly from gradually getting into better alignment while moving your joints through broader ranges of motion.

1. From the Spiderman position, fully straighten the arm next to your lead leg, as shown in Figure 10-4a.

2. While looking at your hand, draw a giant circle by bringing the arm straight overhead in a circular motion, as shown in Figure 10-4b.

3. Continue in a circular motion, bend the elbow, and place the knuckles of your hand on your lower back, as shown in Figure 10-4c, and then reverse the movement.

An essential part of flexibility is relaxation. Try doing these mobility exercises a bit slower than usual, so you can breathe better, feel the movement, and avoid unnecessary tension.

A frames

A frames stretch your calves and hamstrings as well as your hip flexors and glutes. This is a challenging movement for most people, but the payoff is big. Here again, progress comes from gradually increasing your range of motion over months and years of practice.

If you're one of the few who can get into these positions from the beginning, focus on holding the positions longer, so you can further develop your strength. Regardless, be patient with yourself and enjoy the progress.

1. From the Spiderman starting position, while keeping both hands flat on the ground, straighten your lead leg while at the same time pulling your toes up by flexing the lead ankle, as shown in Figure 10-5a.

2. Reset to the Spiderman starting position and lower your left forearm to the ground, as shown in Figure 10-5b.

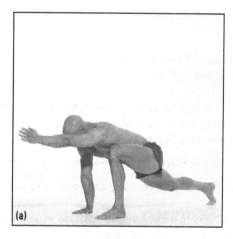
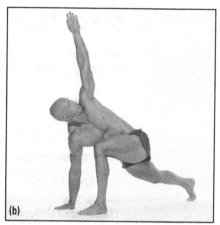
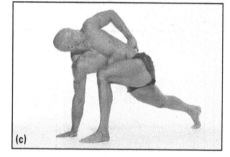

Photo by Jorge Alvarez, www.alvarezphoto.com

FIGURE 10-4:
Arm circles
improve spinal
rotation and
overall shoulder
mobility.

Once you're able to full straighten your lead leg, you can further increase the flex-ibility of your hamstrings by working to straighten your back. Straightening your back causes your pelvis to tilt forward, which pulls on your hamstrings.

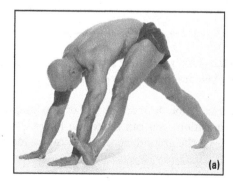
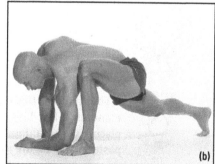

FIGURE 10-5:
Straighten the
lead leg and pull
your toes up (a)
and then reset to
the starting
position and
lower your
forearm (b).

Photo by Jorge Alvarez, www.alvarezphoto.com

Saxon tilts

The Saxon tilt improves lateral flexion and extension of spine, while also challenging your hip and shoulder mobility.

1. After getting into the Spiderman starting position, raise your arms straight overhead while flexing your abdominals, as if you're about to dive into a pool, as shown in Figure 10-6a.

2. Tilt toward the side of your lead leg, as shown in Figure 10-6b.

3. Then tilt toward the side of your rear leg, as shown in Figure 10-6c.

Throughout this exercise, stay in a low lunging position while making yourself tall by fully extending through your arms and fingertips.

FIGURE 10-6:
For the Saxon tilt,
stay in a low
lunging position
while tilting to the
left and right.

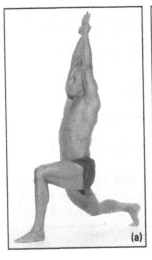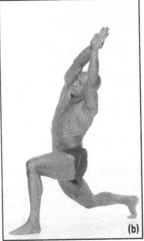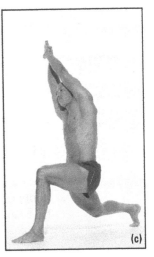

(a) (b) (c)

Photo by Jorge Alvarez, www.alvarezphoto.com

WARNING

This exercise requires a fairly high degree of strength and flexibility. Before doing this exercise, ensure that you are thoroughly warmed up.

TIP

If you find that this exercise is too difficult for you or you simply get too tired to maintain a low lunging position, you can make the lunge quite a bit easier by placing your trailing knee on the ground, so that you're in a long single kneeling position (see Figure 10-7).

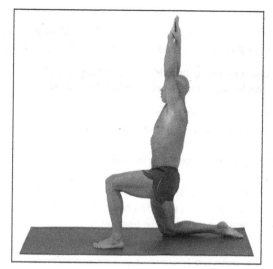

Photo by Mark Lauren

Doing the Inch Worm Exercises

The inch worm exercises start in a push-up position and require you to walk your hands back toward your feet in order to get into various positions, such as a squat or lunge. These movements help strengthen your upper body and core while also improving the strength and flexibility of your lower body.

Bloomers

Bloomers lengthen and strengthen your hamstrings and spinal erectors.

1. **Get into a push-up position with your feet hip width apart, as shown in Figure 10-8a.**

2. **While keeping your legs straight, walk your hands back toward your feet, as shown in Figure 10-8b.**

3. **Once you've walked your hands back to your feet, relax and let your upper body hang over your feet, as shown in Figure 10-8c.**

   Get a good stretch in your hamstrings and relax your neck to let your head hang freely.

4. **Suck your belly button in toward your spine and slowly roll yourself up while continuing to let your head hang freely, as shown in Figure 10-8d.**

5. **Once you're in a standing position, perform a giant arm swing until your arms are straight overhead, as shown in Figure 10-8e.**

   Exhale and make yourself as tall as possible, before completely reversing the movement until you're back in a push-up position.

Typically, when we exercise, we want to maintain a straight back, because that's the safest and most effective position for most activities. However, we also want to learn to control less than ideal positions, because in real life there will be times that we have to do things with a rounded back. Bloomers develop the mobility and stability needed to better control those positions.

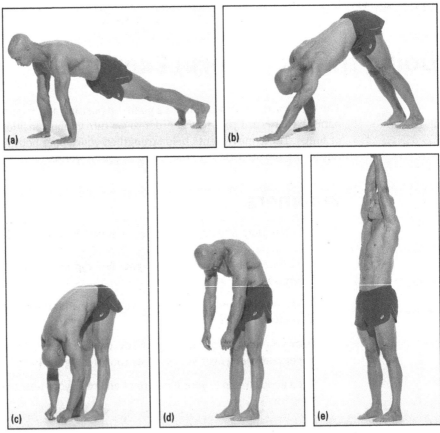

FIGURE 10-8: The bloomer exercise.

Photo by Jorge Alvarez, www.alvarezphoto.com

Take your time as you perform this movement so you can focus on relaxation and control, especially as you roll yourself up and down, since you'll be in a slightly vulnerable position with a rounded back.

Deep squats

This is an incredible exercise for strengthening your entire body while seriously improving ankle mobility.

1. **Get into a push-up position with your feet hip width apart, as shown in Figure 10-9a.**

2. **With a straight back, walk your hips back toward your feet, while bending your knees, as shown in Figure 10-9b.**

3. **Continue to walk your hips back until you're in a squatting position, as shown in Figure 10-9c.**

   In this bottom position of a squat, lift your chest and keep your toes and knees pointed straight ahead.

4. **Stand up tall and straight, as shown in Figure 10-9d, and then reverse the movement until you're back in the starting position.**

To get the most out of this movement, lift your chest in the bottom of the squat. This will do a lot to improve your posture. Also, keep your feet hip width apart with your knees and toes pointed straight ahead. This improves your ankle mobility.

When squatting for the sake of exercise, keep your toes and knees pointing straight ahead. Doing so improves ankle mobility while ingraining the useful habit of keeping your hips neutrally rotated, which means your hips are not externally or internally rotated — they are in the middle. Neutrally rotated hips let you do important activities in your life, such as walk and run, with greater efficiency and safety, because your knees and toes are pointing in the direction that you're going.

Vertical twists

The vertical twist challenges spinal rotation while in a long lunging position, which is great for both full body strength and flexibility.

1. **Get into a stable push-up position, as shown in Figure 10-10a.**

2. **Walk your right leg back until your left knee is directly over your left ankle, as shown in Figure 10-10b.**

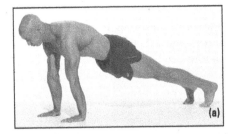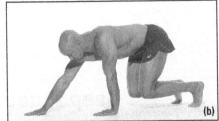
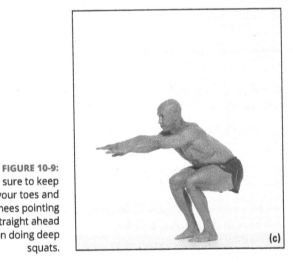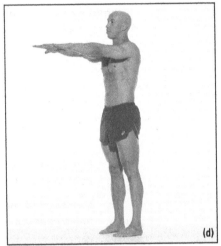

FIGURE 10-9: Be sure to keep your toes and knees pointing straight ahead when doing deep squats.

3. Come to an upright position with your torso and raise your arms directly overhead, as shown in Figure 10-10c.

4. Twist to the left by pulling the left by pulling the left shoulder blade back, as shown in Figure 10-10d.

5. Twist to the right by pulling the right shoulder blade back, as shown in Figure 10-10e.

Throughout this movement, stay in a low lunging position with your abdominals tight and the knee of your trailing knee pointing straight down at the ground. This will train your hip flexors to do their job in a fully lengthened position, while strengthening important postural muscles.

TIP

You can make this exercise easier by placing your trailing knee on the ground, so that you're performing the twisting movement from a long single kneeling position, as shown in Figure 10-11.

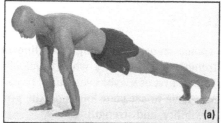 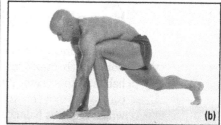

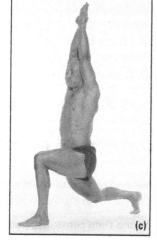 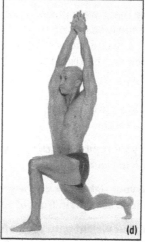 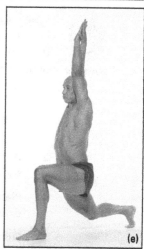

FIGURE 10-10:
The vertical twist builds full body strength and flexibility.

Photo by Jorge Alvarez, www.alvarezphoto.com

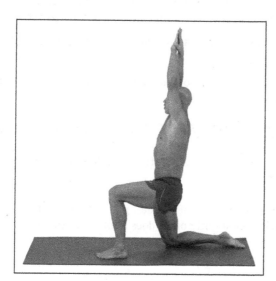

FIGURE 10-11:
Place your knee on the ground to make the vertical twist easier.

Photo by Mark Lauren

Kneeling switches

The kneeling switch is a transition between a single kneeling and squatting position, which improves strength and flexibility while developing useful postural habits. If this seems difficult at first or maybe even hurts, be patient, and focus on controlled movements. You have to set your knees on the ground with control, which requires balance, flexibility, and strength.

REMEMBER

Knees were made were made for kneeling! Getting up and down off the ground is one of the most basic and important athletic skills we possess. More than anything else, a useful indicator of overall fitness is the quality of your joint functions, which can be tested using the floor exercises, as well as your transitions between the lying, kneeling, and standing positions.

1. **Start in a push-up position with your feet hip width apart, as shown in Figure 10-12a.**

2. **Walk your right leg back until your left knee is over your left foot, as shown in Figure 10-12b.**

3. **Place your right knee on the ground and raise your chest with your arms extended straight in front of you, as shown in Figure 10-12c.**

4. **Shift your weight onto your left leg and then climb into a squatting position, as shown in Figure 10-12d.**

   Only the rear leg should move. Challenge yourself to keep all other parts of your body still while switching from a kneeling position to a squat.

5. **Stand up tall and straight, as shown in Figure 10-12e, and then reverse the movement.**

6. **Drop into a squat, switch to a single kneeling position, and walk yourself back out to a planking position.**

When you're in the single kneeling position, before transitioning to a squat, push your hips back slightly so that your upper body has a slight forward tilt, as shown in Figure 10-12c. Also, consciously shift your weight onto the lead leg before stepping in to or out of the squat.

TIP

Anytime you're in the bottom of a squat, get into the habit of lifting your chest. Lifting your chest just slightly often does a lot to fix the most common postural problem, which is a forward head position. The incorrect positioning of the head is mainly the result of being slouched forward at the chest area.

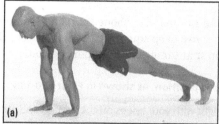
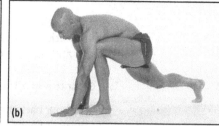
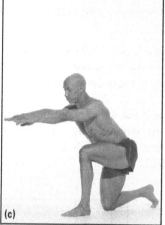
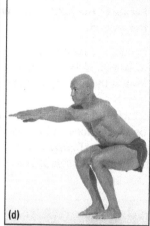
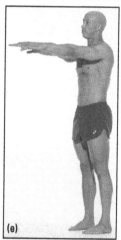

FIGURE 10-12: The kneeling switch is a transition between a single kneeling and squatting position.

Photo by Jorge Alvarez, www.alvarezphoto.com

Mastering the Quadruped Exercises

This is a progression of four movements that starts simple and gradually builds in complexity. Start with the first exercise and move on to the next exercise in the series only once you've mastered the previous exercises.

Kickouts strengthen and lengthen your entire body in a way that is highly useful in day-to-day life, because you are rotating fully around your hips, spine, and shoulders, which evens out the tension surrounding those joints, thereby helping to stabilize them. These movements also develop contralateral (cross-body) hip and shoulder stability by strengthening the connections between your left hip and right shoulder and vice versa, which is important to common activities, such as walking, running, and throwing.

Kickouts

With this movement, you're transitioning between a quadruped and kickout position. The quadruped position is similar to a crawling position, except that your knees are slightly off the ground and about six inches behind your hands. The kickout position is similar to a deep squatting position, except that one leg is fully extended and the arm on that same side is supporting you.

1. **Get into a quadruped position, as shown in Figure 10-13a.**

   Keep your back straight with your knees off the ground and about six inches from your hands.

2. **Rotate to the right slowly while raising your right hand and left foot off the ground.**

   Continue to rotate and pull your left leg underneath yourself until you're able to extend it fully to the kickout position, as shown in Figure 10-13b. Then reverse the movement and reset to the quadruped position.

In the kickout position, fully extend the leg while pulling your toes back toward your body. The toes and knees of the extended leg should be pointing straight up. Lift your chest slightly and let your hips sink down and forward so that you're resting your hips on supporting leg.

FIGURE 10-13:
Quadruped
position (a) to
the kickout
position (b).

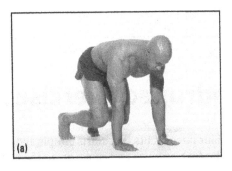 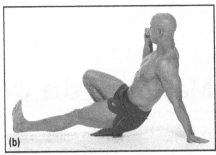

Photo by Jorge Alvarez, www.alvarezphoto.com

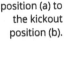

TIP

Kickouts are easier if your knees are close to your hands in the quadruped position. After every kickout, as you reset to quadruped, take the time to position your feet properly so that your knees don't slide farther away from your hands with every rep.

High kicks

This exercise builds on the kickout while also preparing you for the next movement in the progression, which is the side kick. For the high kick, you can expect to feel a strong stretch in your hamstrings, so make sure you're warmed up.

1. Get into a quadruped position, as shown in Figure 10-14a.

2. Rotate to the right and perform a kickout with the left leg, as shown in Figure 10-14b.

3. Reset to the starting position and then straighten your right leg while pushing your chest down toward your feet and kicking your left leg straight up, as shown in Figure 10-14c.

4. Lower yourself to the quadruped position to prepare for the next rep.

As mentioned, you'll likely experience a strong stretch in the hamstring of the supporting leg as you perform the high kick, so take your time. If you want more of a stretch, fully straighten the supporting leg, keep the foot flat on the ground, and straighten your back while pushing your chest toward your feet.

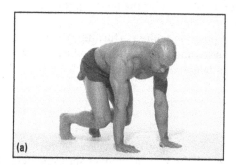

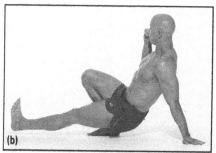

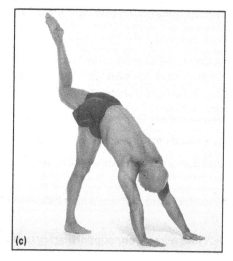

FIGURE 10-14: The high kick produces a strong stretch in your hamstrings.

Photo by Jorge Alvarez, www.alvarezphoto.com

Side kicks

This side kick stretches the side of your body and prepares you for the next movement in this series, which is the table top.

1. Get into the quadruped starting position, as shown in Figure 10-15a.
2. Perform a kickout with the left leg, as shown in Figure 10-15b.
3. Reset to the starting position and kick the left leg straight up, as shown in Figure 10-15c, while fully extending the supporting leg and pushing your chest down toward your feet.
4. From the high kick position, reach across your body to the right side with your left leg, as shown in Figure 10-15d.
5. Once you feel a stretch along the left side of your body, return to the quadruped position to prepare for the next repetition.

Make yourself as tall as possible while performing the side kick by keeping the supporting leg fully extended and your chest pushed down toward your feet. Making yourself tall will challenge and improve your hamstring, hip, and shoulder mobility.

Table tops

This is the final movement in the four movement series of kickout exercises. Each movement in this progression builds on the previous one to bring you to this final point — the table top.

In addition to all the benefits of the previous movements, the table top seriously improves spinal rotation while strengthening and lengthening your entire body. It's a relatively difficult movement so be patient and don't rush the progression. Also, make sure you're warmed up.

1. Start in a relaxed quadruped position, as shown in Figure 10-16a.
2. Rotate to the right and perform a kickout with the left leg, as shown in Figure 10-16b.
3. Reset to the starting position and perform a high kick with the left leg, as shown in Figure 10-16c.
4. Bring the elevated left foot across your supporting leg to the right, as shown in Figure 10-16d.
5. Continue to reach across your body with your left leg until your left hand comes off the ground, and then place your left foot on the ground next to your right foot while reaching straight up with the left arm, as shown in Figure 10-16e.

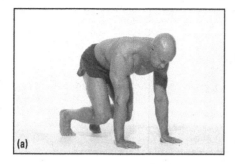
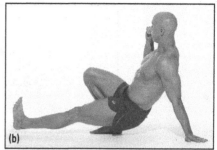
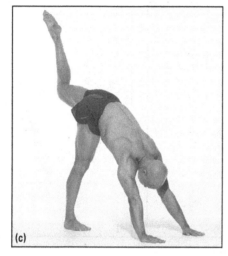
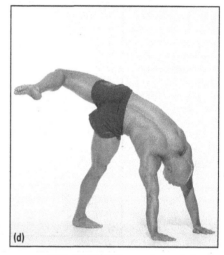

FIGURE 10-15: The side kick stretches the side of your body.

Photo by Jorge Alvarez, www.alvarezphoto.com

The table top exercise requires awareness of where your limbs are in space relative to one another, and because the movement requires this skill, it also helps to develop it. It takes practice and experience to position yourself properly. In the end position, your feet should be about shoulder width apart, with your knees and toes pointing in the same direction. Raise your hips and create a straight vertical line with your arms.

TIP

This exercise is significantly easier if you keep your hips low during the transition from high kick to table top. If you really want to challenge your mobility, perform a proper high kick and side kick with your hips fully elevated, and then transition to table tops while keeping your hips up. With that said, it's totally okay to make the exercise easier by keeping your hips low, if needed. You can then progress the movement by gradually increasing the height of your hips. As always, listen to your body and don't push to the point of pain.

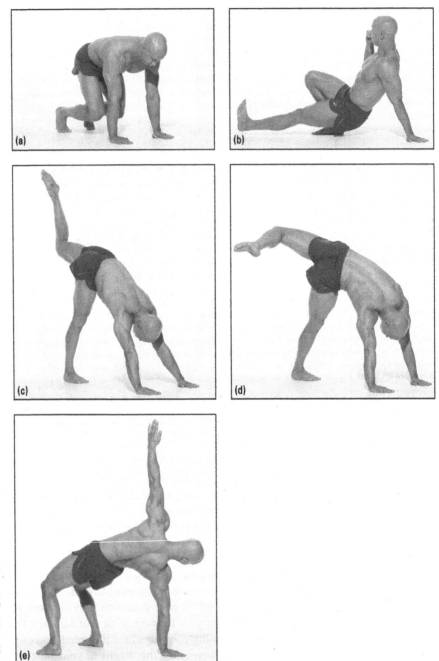

FIGURE 10-16:
The table top is the result of the progression of the previous three exercises, and the most difficult.

Trying the Starfish Exercises

This series is a progression of four movements that improve hip, core, and upper body strength while teaching you to move your hips and shoulders independent of one another, so you can rotate better.

Strengthening your core while improving rotation around the spine has a big carryover to real life activities. Think about it for a second . . . how many activities require rotation? Almost anytime that there is a weight shift, spinal rotation is involved. Some examples of that are walking, running, throwing, punching, kicking, swimming, golfing, bowling, and so on.

Starfish twists

The main purpose of this movement is to strengthen the sides of your body (your external obliques) while improving spinal rotation.

1. **Get into the starting position of a push-up with your feet hip width apart, as shown in Figure 10-17a. Your shoulders should be directly over your wrists.**

2. **Rotate your body to the left and raise your right arm straight overhead, as shown in Figure 10-17b.**

    You should be on the sides of your feet with your heels on the ground.

3. **While keeping the right arm up, rotate your hips fully to the right, as shown in Figure 10-17c.**

4. **Once you've fully rotated your hips, bring the right arm down and return to a long straight push-up position.**

The key to getting the most out of these Starfish exercises is to make yourself as long and straight as possible in all positions. Doing so requires paying attention to your entire body and developing a feel for where you are in space.

REMEMBER

If you have problems with wrist pain, try doing this exercise on a hard surface. Using a soft mat to support your hands increases the bend in your wrists and can therefore aggravate them.

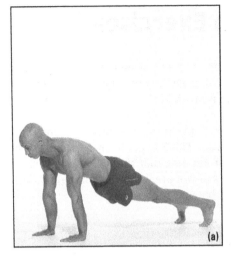
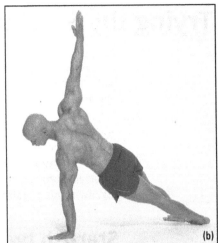

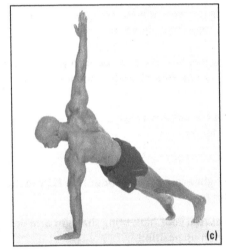

FIGURE 10-17: Starfish twists help strengthen your external obliques.

REMEMBER

Learning to make yourself long and straight in a wide variety of situations, such as standing, kneeling, lying positions, side planking, and so on, has an incredibly useful carryover to real-life activities and sports. Making yourself long and straight means finding the middle (you aren't tall if you're bent in any direction). Knowing where the middle is gives you a good reference point for knowing where you are in space. Additionally, your joints are safest when they are in the middle, meaning neutrally aligned. In contrast, your joints are most vulnerable when they are at their extreme ranges of motion.

Starfish hip drops

The starfish hip drop builds on the starfish twist by adding lateral flexion and extension to the movement, which strengthens and lengthens the sides of your body.

1. Start in a push-up position with your feet hip width apart, as shown in Figure 10-18a.

2. Rotate fully onto your left side, as shown in Figure 10-18b, and raise your right arm overhead.

3. While keeping your supporting arm straight and your elevated arm pointing straight up, lower your hips to the ground, as shown in Figure 10-18c. Then raise your hips again until you're straight from head to heels.

4. While keeping the right arm up, rotate your hips fully, as shown in Figure 10-18d.

5. After fully rotating your hips, place your right hand on the ground again and return to a planking position.

If you can't lower your hips all the way to the ground, as described in Step 3, simply lower your hips as far as you comfortably can. As you progress, you'll be able to increase your range of motion until you're able to lower your hips all the way to the ground.

Starfish push-ups

This exercise builds on the starfish twist by adding a push-up to the end of the movement, which strengthens your chest, shoulders, triceps, forearms, and core.

1. Get into a push-up position with your feet hip width apart, as shown in Figure 10-19a.

2. Transition to a side planking position on your left side with your right arm reaching to the sky, as shown in Figure 10-19b.

3. Rotate your hips to the right without moving the elevated arm, as shown in Figure 10-19c.

4. After fully rotating the hips, place your right hand on the ground and drop into the bottom of a push-up, as shown in Figure 10-19d.

5. Press yourself back up to the starting position of a push-up to complete the rep.

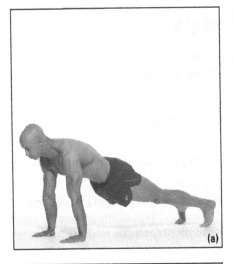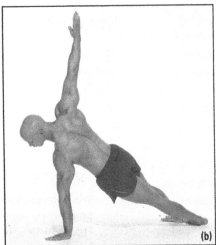

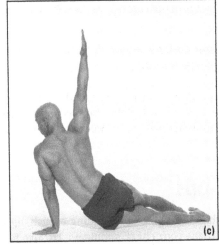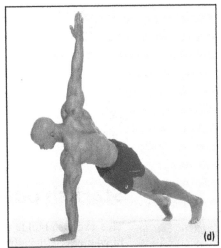

Photo by Jorge Alvarez, www.alvarezphoto.com

FIGURE 10-18: The starfish hip drop builds on the starfish twist by adding lateral flexion and extension.

They key here is to perform all parts of this movement while keeping yourself straight from head to toe. Keep your hips in the middle and your head aligned.

TIP

If you can't do a push-up, no problem. Simply lower yourself to the bottom of a push-up with as much control as possible, and then "cheat" yourself back up however you can. This is a great technique for developing strength with difficult movements. If an exercise is too hard for you, start by learning to control the downward portion of the movement, and then "cheat" yourself back into position for the next rep.

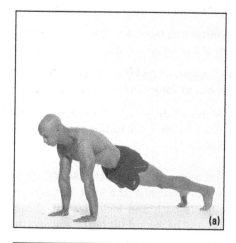 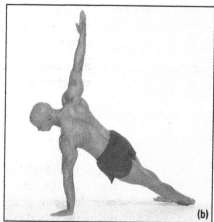

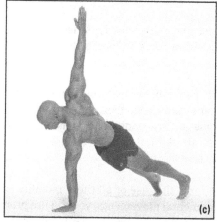 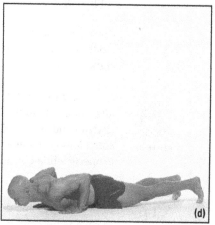

FIGURE 10-19: The starfish push-up builds on the starfish twist by adding a push-up to the end of the movement.

Photo by Jorge Alvarez, www.alvarezphoto.com

Starfish dive bombers

This exercise builds on the starfish push-up by adding a seesaw type movement to the bottom of the push-up once you're lying flat on the ground. The main purpose of this movement is to improve spinal extension and front to back tilting of your shoulder blades, which will improve your posture.

1. Get into a push-up position, as shown in Figure 10-20a.

2. Shift your weight to the left and fully rotate onto your left side, as shown in Figure 10-20b.

3. While keeping your right arm reaching straight up, rotate your hips to the right, as shown in Figure 10-20c.

4. After fully rotating your hips, place your right hand on the ground and drop into the bottom of a push-up, as shown in Figure 10-2od.

5. Place both knees on the ground and then lift your chest off the ground by straightening your arms, as shown in Figure 10-2oe.

6. While keeping your knees on the ground, bend your elbows and lower your chest between your hands while raising your hips into the air, as shown in Figure 10-2of.

As you straighten your arms and raise your chest in Step 5, try to relax and let your hips sink into the ground to maximize the stretch. Once your arms are fully extended, pull your shoulders back and look straight ahead. This position is where the spinal extension and backward tilt of the *scapula* (the shoulder blades) comes from.

Once you lower your chest and raise your hips, let your shoulders tilt forward slightly in the bottom position. This is where the forward tilt of the scapula comes from.

REMEMBER

Good posture isn't a static position, because you're not a static object. Ideal joint alignment is fluid and situation dependent, which is why it requires a bit of rhythm and special awareness. These mobility exercises are dynamic for that reason, so you can develop the strength, flexibility, and awareness needed to position properly while constantly transitioning.

TIP

If you want exercise programs that use of all these mobility exercises, including floor exercises and developmental movements, you can use promo code STRONG15 to save 15 percent on annual memberships at marklauren.com.

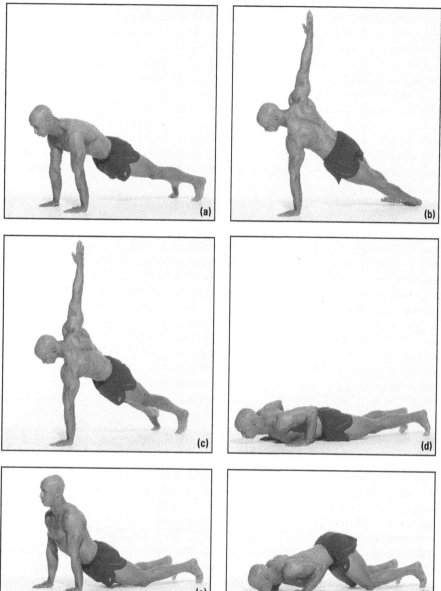

FIGURE 10-20: The purpose of dive bombers is to improve spinal extension and front to back tilting of your shoulder blades.

Photo by Jorge Alvarez, www.alvarezphoto.com

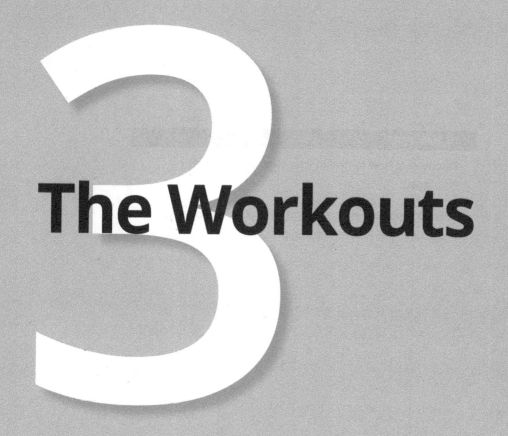

The Workouts

3

Discovering how to design your workouts to meet your goals.

Following specific exercises and workouts, day by day, in the ultimate 13-week fitness program.

IN THIS CHAPTER

» Choosing exercises to meet your current goals

» Focusing your training effort with training splits

» Adapting your workouts for long-term progress

» Covering the essentials to avoid injury

» Allowing time for active recovery

Chapter **11**

Mixing and Matching Exercises for Your Goals

While this book gives you all the tools you to need to achieve your fitness goals, only you can achieve your personal goals — by understanding and then customizing exactly which exercises and workouts you need.

Choosing Your Workout Types

The needs of newbies are different from those of intermediate and advanced users. No matter what level you are at, over time, your life changes, you change, and your fitness goals will change as well. Equipped with this chapter's knowledge, you will be able to combine exercises into different types of workouts to apply stress to your muscles in targeted ways and achieve specific objectives.

In order to optimize your gains and minimize the risk of injury, stress from exercise should be applied thoughtfully and with structure. As a general rule, just enough is enough. Listen to your body. Overdoing it can slow progress and lead to injury.

The following workout types refer mainly to the way repetitions are combined to create sets. A full workout can consist of a single workout type that's repeated, or multiple ones combined.

Sets across

This is when you perform the same exercise for the same number of reps in multiple sets and is probably the simplest and most common workout. An example of sets across is doing three sets of 12 repetitions of push-ups. The benefit of using sets across is that it's a very simple way to adjust training volume. For example, a beginner might do just one set of 12 repetitions, while a more advanced user might do four sets of 12 repetitions.

Using sets across, you can systematically progress by increasing the number of reps per set and/or by increasing the total number of sets. For example, you could progress from doing two sets of 8 reps to doing two sets of 12 reps. You could also progress from doing two sets of eight reps to doing four sets of eight reps. Both examples start with a total number of 16 reps and end with a total number of 24 reps, but you've arrived at the increase of total reps in different ways.

Additionally, you can adjust the rest intervals between sets to shift the training focus between strength and endurance. Somewhat oversimplified, more rest between sets allows for greater strength, whereas less rest between sets shifts the emphasis to endurance.

Supersets

Supersets are when you perform two exercises back-to-back without rest. The two exercises should complement each other by stressing overlapping muscles.

An example of a superset is doing 12 repetitions of squats, and then immediately after, executing 12 reps of glute hip-ups. Squats work all your leg muscles, while hip-ups focus in on your glutes.

TIP

Supersets develop both strength and endurance by adding intensity and variety while improving blood flow to the muscles (known as "the pump").

There's plenty of room for creativity and experimentation since there's endless ways to pair exercises. With that said, my favorite technique for supersets is to combine the floor exercises from Chapter 4 with pushing, pulling, leg, or core exercises. The floor exercises prepare you for better positioning with more complex movements.

These exercise combinations don't need to be intentional or based on improving movement quality. Random combinations are also a useful and fun way to learn. It's often interesting seeing how muscles and body parts are connected by performing different movement combinations.

Ladders

Ladders are a great way to develop muscular endurance and strength with high volume, low intensity training. They give you relatively easy practice in the lower rep ranges, typically between one and seven. Strength is gained through repetition, like anything else, which is why doing a lot of low repetition sets is so useful — you get plenty of practice in a short amount of time, which also improves endurance.

To perform a ladder, start by choosing an exercise. Then do one rep followed by a brief moment of rest. Then do two reps followed by a slightly longer rest period. Then perform three reps followed by a slightly longer rest period. You can go up the "ladder" as high as you want, but keep in mind that you need to come back down the ladder in the same manner. Ideally, you want to come back down from the ladder early enough that you avoid hitting muscle failure.

Here's an example of a ladder going up to four repetitions:

>> One rep and five seconds of rest

>> Two reps and ten seconds of rest

>> Three reps and 15 seconds of rest

>> Four reps and 20 seconds of rest

>> Three reps and 15 seconds of rest

>> Two reps and ten seconds of rest

>> One rep and five seconds of rest

You could also repeatedly go up and down the ladder, maybe up to six reps the first time and only up to four reps the second time. The possibilities are endless. Take a playful approach and keep it easy.

TIP

If you want exact rep-to-rep and day-to-day guidance, see me at marklauren. com where I have years of well-thought-out programs that progress from beginner to advanced levels. Use promo code STRONG15 to save 15 percent on annual memberships.

Timed sets

Timed sets are a great tool for bodyweight exercises, because they allow users of varying fitness levels to get equally beneficial workouts using the same exercises. You simply choose the work and rest intervals, as well as the total number of sets to be completed.

For example, you could do three sets using 40-second work intervals and 20-second rest intervals. That means that you would exercise for 40 seconds and then rest for 20 seconds before starting the next set. The intention is to perform as many clean reps as possible in each work interval. It's okay to take mini-breaks in order to avoid complete muscle failure, so you're not completely useless for the rest of the set and remainder of the workout.

Using the same exercise and work intervals, a novice trainee might do five reps per set while a more advanced trainee might do 15 reps per set. Both users challenge themselves successfully using the exact same workout.

Speed sets

There is a strong correlation between strength and speed. Improving speed usually results in improved strength and vice versa.

For speed sets, you choose an exercise that you can do for about 8 to 12 repetitions. You then perform eight to ten sets of two-three reps with short 15-30 seconds rest periods between sets. During each repetition, focus on explosive upward movements and perfect form. This training technique develops explosive power, strength, and size. It's a great way to blast through plateaus.

Here's an example of a speed set: Find a variation of push-ups (maybe with your hands elevated on a counter top) that you can do 8 to 12 times, and then do three explosive repetitions every 15 seconds for a total of ten sets. That's ten sets of three repetitions using 15-second rest intervals.

Speed sets work very well with plyometric type movements like Iron Mikes or dynamic squats, because these movements inherently require speed to get you off the ground. You also don't want to do plyometrics to the point where your form deteriorates, which is why frequent, low-rep sets with short rest intervals work so well.

Circuit training

Circuit training involves performing a series of different exercises in sequence, usually with minimal rest. Circuit training can be combined with timed sets, whereby users perform the exercises for set work intervals and then use the rest intervals to transition to the next exercise.

This method of training allows for endless variety and can easily be tailored to various fitness levels and goals. It's also an easy way to build full body workouts that develop both strength and cardiovascular endurance.

A circuit training workout with eight exercises can accommodate up to 24 people who rotate between exercises without getting in each other's way. This is especially applicable when equipment is being used, like pull-up bars or dip bars.

Consider this example of full body circuit training: Complete three rounds of the following exercises using 40-second work intervals and 20-second rest intervals:

>> Dynamic squats (legs)

>> Modified push-ups (pushing)

>> Let-me-ins (pulling)

>> Starfish crunches (core)

For this example, the user would do as many perfect reps of each exercise as possible in 40 seconds, and then transition to the next exercise during the 20-second rest intervals.

With circuit training, the options are endless.

Flows

Commonly used by yoga practitioners, *flows* are sequences of movements linked in a smooth and continuous manner. The transitions between positions or exercises are fluid and intentional, with a strong focus on maintaining ideal alignment and positioning at all times, including during the transition between exercises. The pace of these workouts is usually slower than other workout types.

The main benefit of flows is learning to move mindfully so that you can improve overall movement quality through greater awareness and coordination. Flows, which are typically mobility based, are an extremely effective complement to more conventional strength training methods. Improving and maintaining mobility is an essential part of building a physique that is both strong and athletic!

Once you begin strength training, flows continue to be exceptionally useful by keeping you athletic as you build strength.

A great way to create flows is to combine movements in the following order:

>> Floor exercises

>> Mobility exercises

>> Kneeling transitions

>> Leg exercises

Flows that are built using this template cover your hip, spine, and shoulder functions (floor exercises), dynamic strength and flexibility (mobility exercises), developmental movements (kneeling transitions), and standing basics, such as squats, lunges, and step-ups (leg exercises).

Here is an example of exercises stacked together to create a flow:

1. Pointer (floor exercise)

2. Starfish twist (mobility exercise)

3. Long kneeling transition

4. Side lunge (leg exercise)

You could do four repetitions on the left side only, and then do four repetitions on the right side. To build an entire workout, you can put together several of these exercise stacks or simply repeat the same stack of exercises.

One of the great things about building flows this way is that you're constantly transitioning between various lying, kneeling, and standing positions, which makes you strong in an incredibly functional way. Additionally, the floor exercises prepare you for the mobility exercises, and the mobility exercises prepare you for better movement quality in the standing positions. Simply put, building flows in this manner creates progressions from simple to complex.

REMEMBER

The quality of your joint functions contribute greatly to your overall fitness. For this reason, it's important to practice flows and routines that have these often ignored basics built into them.

Focusing Your Training with Training Splits

When you exercise, you're applying stress to your body with the intention of bringing about positive results. However, if that stress is not applied strategically, your progress could slow, halt, or reverse, making you weaker instead of stronger.

One of the best ways to control and target exercise stress is to decide which *training split* you'll use, which basically means determining which parts of your body are targeted in a single workout. There are many types of training splits, but for the purpose of bodyweight exercises, the choices are these:

» Full body workouts

» Upper and lower body workouts

» Pushing, pulling, legs, and core workouts

Simply put, there is a progression from a broad distribution of stress throughout the entire body to a more focused and targeted application of stress. The following sections cover what you need to know about each of these training splits.

Full body workouts

Full body routines evenly distribute the stress of a training session by using movements from each of the main movement categories — pushing, pulling, legs, and core. For most people, the even distribution of stress is enough to stimulate adaptations. Unless you're an advanced user, applying stress to isolated body parts or regions simply isn't necessary.

With full body workouts, you can stimulate your entire body three times a week with just three workouts. If full body workouts are enough to spur the progress you want, stimulating the entire body three times a week is better than just once a week through a more isolated split.

Additionally, full body workouts duplicate the stress of real life and sports. When you're working on a farm, moving furniture, playing with your kids, or doing most anything else, your entire body is involved. Full body workouts encourage symmetrical and balanced development, along with a stronger metabolic response and calorie burn. I also believe that even distribution of stress over the entire body improves movement quality and longevity.

Start with full body workouts and then progresses to upper and lower body splits and finally to workouts isolated to pushing, pulling, legs, and core.

REMEMBER

A simple and timeless training split that works for countless athletes and fitness enthusiasts is to do a full body training split with workouts on Mondays, Wednesdays, and Fridays. Don't be seduced by fancy fads. Keep it simple and vary your training by using different exercise variations and workout types.

Upper and lower body workouts

Upper and lower body training splits cover the entire body in two training sessions. The upper body workout combines pushing and pulling exercises, while the lower body workout combines leg and core exercises. Core movements are included in lower body because the hips are part of your core.

Quality workouts require only four exercises per session, not including warm up and cool down. While full body workouts can include one exercise for pushing, pulling, legs, and core (four total exercises), upper body workouts use two pushing and two pulling movements to double the amount of stress on the upper body when compared to a full body workout. Likewise, a lower body workout doubles the stress on the lower body by using two movements for the legs and two movements for the core.

>> An upper body workout might look something like this: Push-ups (push), let-me-ins (pull), military presses (push), and let-me-ups (pull).

>> A lower body workout might be: Squats (legs), hanging leg lifts (core), lunges (legs), and reverse hypers (core).

Applying more stress to your upper or lower body requires more recovery time, which you get because you don't do back-to-back upper body workouts or back-to-back lower body workouts. An appropriate training split could be as follows:

>> Monday: Upper body

>> Tuesday: Lower body

>> Wednesday: Rest

>> Thursday: Upper body

>> Friday: Lower body

In this example, you're training the entire body twice a week.

Pushing, pulling, legs, and core workouts

In this training split, four exercises from the same movement category make up a single workout. Pushing workouts have four pushing movements. Pulling workouts have four pulling movements, and so on. The exercise stress on the targeted area is doubled from the previous training split.

REMEMBER

Full body workouts use just one exercise from each movement category. Upper and lower body workouts use two exercises from each movement category, and this training split uses four movements from each category.

Your overall fitness and age determine what is appropriate for you. Be ready to change and adapt as needed. What worked for you last year or last month might not work for you now. If you are diligent and consistent, you will need more, which might mean bigger full body workouts or a more isolated training split.

Adapting Your Workouts for Long-Term Progress

Fitness, like other things in life, tends to flow in waves and cycles. Your training should progress in cycles that enable you to take two or three steps forward and then back off a step to allow for full recovery. It's unrealistic to expect endless linear progress. Recognize the value of rest and recuperation and adapt your training accordingly.

Volume and intensity

Simply put, there are two variables that you can adjust when training: volume and intensity.

>> *Volume* refers to how much you're doing. In the case of calisthenics, it refers to the total number of repetitions in a workout.

>> *Intensity* refers to the difficulty of each movement. For example, push-ups with your hands elevated on a countertop are less intense than push-ups with your hands on the ground.

REMEMBER

Generally speaking, as training volume increases training intensity decreases. When it comes to exercise, it makes sense to do more of something when it's easy and less of it when it's difficult.

For complete beginners, volume and intensity should both be low. Progress your workouts to higher volume while keeping intensity low. Once you achieve a relatively high level of training volume over the course of several weeks or months, decrease the volume and increase the difficulty of the exercises.

Using adjustments in training volume and intensity, you can optimize these cyclical programs for long-term progress. This is why training routines are often referred to as training *cycles*. A training cycle is typically anywhere from two to six weeks.

TIP

I have a strong preference for full body splits, where you train your entire body three times per week on Mondays, Wednesdays, and Fridays. One very important reason that I prefer this training split is because it's easy to adjust volume and intensity. As a person advances, more and more stress is needed to make further progress, which means more recovery time will also be needed. At some point, you won't have enough time to recover from three full body workouts per week. At that point, the volume of Wednesday's workout can simply be reduced to allow for full recovery by Friday. Likewise, about once a month, volume and intensity can be reduced for all workouts within a week to allow for an active recovery week, which we talk about shortly.

Consistency and variety

To make meaningful and measurable progress, you should be consistent. Stick with a routine for a while in order to make progress, before switching. You can apply training cycles to focus on different skills and qualities, such as strength, speed, and endurance. Trying to improve everything at once simply doesn't work. You need to focus and stay consistent. With that said, you also can't do the exact same thing over and over. Change causes adaptation. You should continuously incorporation little variations into your workouts.

Play around with exercise variations, workout types, number of sets and reps, and rest periods. It's not too different from academic learning — you won't become better by writing the exact same thing over and over or by solving the same math problem again and again.

Progression and regression

Good routines make forward progress by increasing volume or intensity, and they back off slightly by decreasing volume or intensity. You need to build active recovery workouts into all your routines. These are workouts with decreased volume and/or intensity. Backing off your training can be hard and counterintuitive, but it can have a very high payoff. You get stronger while you rest — and you decrease your chances of injury.

That's why the 13-week training plan in this book has an active recovery week at the end of the program (see Chapter 12).

Covering the Essentials to Avoid Injury

Your well-being and physical performance depend on the strength of your foundation, which is made up of fundamental movement skills. These are the essentials that are used in every movement, and that's why the basics are so extremely valuable! First in the list of athletic essentials are joint functions. Next are the transitions between lying, kneeling, and standing positions, which involve controlled weight shifting with coordinated hip and shoulder movements.

Joint functions and transitions

As mentioned, these are used all the time, including during your workouts. To prepare yourself for long-term success, ensure that the basics are in place by practicing the exercises in Chapters 4 and 5. They allow for better progress without annoying setbacks and avoidable injuries.

Beginning with warm ups

The floor exercises are made up of four exercise categories for back lying, side lying, front lying, and crawling movements. Each of these categories in turn has four exercises. A great warmup is to do four to eight repetitions with the exercises from one of the categories. Use a different category each training day.

TIP

If you find the floor exercises too difficult for a warm up, do three sets of marching in place with 40-second work intervals and 20-second rest intervals. You can also do 60 seconds of marching in place before doing the floor exercises.

Wrapping up with cool downs

A great time to practice your developmental movements is at the end of your training session, as your cool down. Pick a movement, like rolling, and practice it. Getting in and out of the kneeling positions is great for your posture, improves balance, and loosens up your hips. It's exactly what you need to recalibrate after a good session.

If those transitions are too hard for you as cool downs, you can simply do some light walking, which is also extremely useful!

Lastly, it's also not a bad idea to lay flat on the ground for a few minutes. It's a simple thing that helps you relax before facing the world again. Try lying on your back with your arms at about the T position with your lower legs elevated on a couch. It's a very relaxing and comfortable position that's great for your back.

Allowing time for active recovery

People often resist slowing down. A lot of people just want to *go, go, go* . . . all the time, and this is true with fitness enthusiasts too! But it is absolutely essential to make time to rest. Especially as you age, one of your biggest challenges may be resisting the urge to do more than is safe. Just enough is enough.

With that said, it's hard to know exactly how much is just right, and for that reason, you might want to put the petal to the metal for only a set period of time, and then back off a bit to allow for full recovery and improved injury resistance. Exercise stress can build up from workout to workout, which is a good thing, *if* you allow time for active recovery. If you don't, it'll lead to suboptimal results, injury, and burnout.

IN THIS CHAPTER

» **Getting familiar with the workouts**

» **Starting with Block 1: Weeks 1-4**

» **Building with Block 2: Weeks 5-8**

» **Maintaining with Block 3: Weeks 9-12**

» **Adding an active recovery week**

Chapter **12**

Following a 13-Week Program

This chapter lays out a 13-week program that is split into three, four-week "blocks" that gradually progress in difficulty. There are six workouts per week that are each fewer than 30 minutes, for a weekly total of 2 to 3 hours. If that's too much time for you, don't worry. You have the option of doing just three workouts per week. More on that later in the chapter.

Mondays, Wednesdays, and Fridays are full body strength training days. Tuesdays, Thursdays, and Saturdays are easier mobility-based workouts that improve your recovery and joint health. If you're limited on time, you can do just the three strength training workouts per week, which also benefit your mobility. Sunday is a rest day. It's important to rest physically and mentally so you will be ready to hit it with gusto again the next day.

Creating a Tailored Routine

These workouts are designed to be as simple and flexible as possible in order to accommodate people of all fitness levels. The strength training workouts allow you to do as many or as few repetitions as you want. An absolute novice will do a low volume of total repetitions, while someone more advanced might double or triple that number. With that said, it's a mistake to place a lot of value on numbers, such as the number or repetitions or rounds you do. It's much better to focus on technique and movement quality. You'll have more fun, get better results, and be more likely to keep showing up.

TIP

Make safety and consistency your priority. Focus on form first and forget about how many reps or rounds you're doing. Especially in the beginning, take as many breaks as you want. This will improve your technique, which decreases your risk of injury while maximizing performance.

Some people might find the movements in the strength training workouts too difficult, and that's okay. For those readers, I recommend doing only the workouts on Tuesdays, Thursdays, and Saturdays, which consist of the floor exercises from Chapter 4, which specifically train all the joint functions of your hips, spine, and shoulders.

After completing a full 13 weeks of those workouts, give the strength training workouts another try. However, if you're getting great results from just the floor exercises, it's not a bad idea to stick with that same routine for another 13 weeks. The goal is to keep progressing for the rest of your life, so there's no rush. If you're making progress, don't make things harder than they need to be. Slow is smooth; smooth is fast.

Introducing the Workouts

There are three types of strength training sessions in this program, all of which are full body workouts — AMRAPs, timed sets, and circuit training.

AMRAPs

For AMRAP (as many rounds as possible) workouts, you perform the exercises back-to-back for a fixed period of time. Each time you complete the given number of reps, you have completed one round. AMRAPs allow you to work at your own pace while developing strength and endurance. These workouts allow you to do a lot of work in a short amount of time, so focus on finding a consistent and sustainable pace throughout the duration of the workout. These sessions are a great way to get your metabolism fired up and improve your body composition.

In the following example, the exercises are to be repeated back-to-back for 16 minutes. For the workouts, we give you brief workout descriptions as well as starting and ending images for all the exercises, along with chapter references to the full descriptions.

AMRAPs: 16 mins

Parallel leg bridges: 12 reps

Zombie squats: 10 reps

Starfish twists: 12 reps

Back lunges: 10 reps

Timed sets

For timed sets, you complete a given number of sets of each exercise, with timed work and rest intervals. Repeatedly doing the same exercise with short rest intervals in between allows you to apply more focused stress to specific parts of your body while still working at your own pace, since there is no designated number of reps during each work interval.

In the following example, try each exercise in four consecutive sets, using 40-second work intervals and 40-second rest intervals, before moving on to the next exercise.

Timed Sets: 4 sets x 40 sec on/ 40 sec off

Bodyrocks

Parallel leg bridges

Let-me-ins or slow swimmers

Dynamic squats

Circuit training

These workouts combine rounds and timed intervals. They allow you to push yourself a bit harder than with timed sets, because you aren't doing the same exercise back-to-back. By rotating through all the exercises with fixed work and rest intervals, you can train at your own pace while distributing the workload of the exercises more evenly.

In the following example, perform a single set of each exercise, using a 40-second work interval and a 20-second rest interval, before moving on to the next exercise. Repeat all the exercises for four rounds.

Circuit Training

Four Rounds — 40 sec on/20 sec off

Parallel leg crunches: 8 reps
Zombie squats: 10 reps
Starfish twists: 8 reps
Skydivers arms at side: 20 reps

Block 1: Weeks 1-4

Now that you have an idea of each of the types of workouts in this 13-week routine, the rest of the chapter breaks the routine into logical, four-week blocks. Each week in Block 1 is the same, so you repeat the training days for four weeks and then move on to Block 2.

TIP

If you find an exercise too difficult, feel free to replace it with an exercise from the same chapter/category. For example, if the bodyrock is too hard, you can replace it with any other core exercise. For personalized assistance and recommendations, use the chat tool at marklauren.com and ask us anything.

Here is an overview of the training days in Block 1:

Monday	Tuesday	Wednesday
Timed Sets	**Back Lying Exercises**	**AMRAP**
Bodyrocks	Dead bugs	Back lunges: 6 reps
Slow swimmers	Glute hip-ups	Tripod scissor kicks: 8 reps
Squats	Windshield wipers	Romanian deadlifts: 6 reps
Glute hip-ups	Up and overs	Y-cuffs: 8 reps

Thursday	Friday	Saturday
Crawling Exercises	**Circuit Training**	**Front Lying Exercises**
Dirty dogs	Parallel leg crunches	Hip twists
Hip circles	T-arm squats	Moose antlers
Straight wide legs	Starfish twists	Twists and reaches
Pointers	Skydivers arms at sides	Y-cuffs

Monday

Monday is all about *timed sets*. Perform three sets of each exercise, using 40-second work intervals and 40-second rest intervals. Alternate sides after each rep for single-sided exercises, like slow swimmers.

Bodyrocks

Figure 12-1 shows the starting and ending positions for the bodyrocks movement. For a full description of this exercise, see Chapter 6.

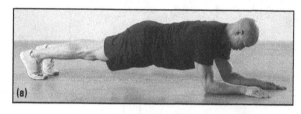
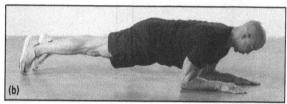

Photo by Jorge Alvarez, www.alvarezphoto.com

FIGURE 12-1: Get into a straight planking position on your forearms (a) and then rock yourself back and forth while staying straight, head to heels (b).

Slow swimmers

Figure 12-2 shows the starting and ending positions for slow swimmers. For a full description of this exercise, see Chapter 6.

Squats

Figure 12-3 shows the starting and ending positions for squats. For a full description of this exercise, see Chapter 7.

Glute hip-ups

Figure 12-4 shows the starting and ending positions for glute hip-ups. Alternate sides after each rep. For a full description of this exercise, see Chapter 4.

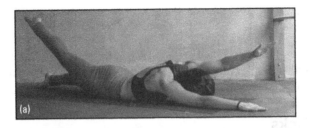
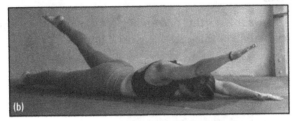

FIGURE 12-2:
Raise your left
arm and right leg
(a) and then raise
your right arm
and left leg (b).

Photo by Jorge Alvarez, www.alvarezphoto.com

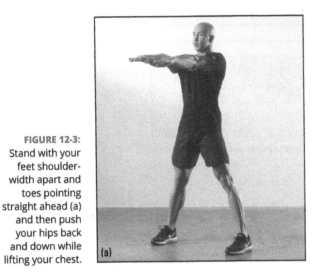
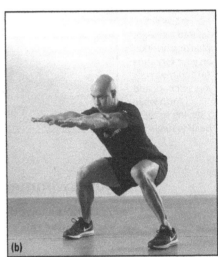

FIGURE 12-3:
Stand with your
feet shoulder-
width apart and
toes pointing
straight ahead (a)
and then push
your hips back
and down while
lifting your chest.

Photo by Jorge Alvarez, www.alvarezphoto.com

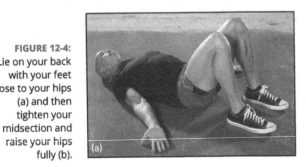
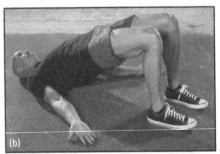

FIGURE 12-4:
Lie on your back
with your feet
close to your hips
(a) and then
tighten your
midsection and
raise your hips
fully (b).

Photo by Jorge Alvarez, www.alvarezphoto.com

Tuesday

Tuesday involves back lying exercises. Perform each exercise for a single set of six repetitions. For single-sided exercises, do all the reps on your left side and then on your right side.

Dead bugs

Figure 12-5 shows the starting and ending positions for dead bugs. For a full description of this exercise, see Chapter 4.

FIGURE 12-5:
Lie on your back with your knees directly over your hips (a) and then extend your left leg fully while pressing your lower back into the ground (b). Repeat with your right leg.

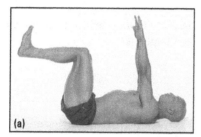 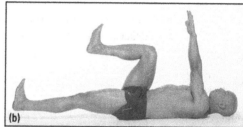

Photo by Jorge Alvarez, www.alvarezphoto.com

Glute hip-ups

Figure 12-6 shows the starting and ending positions for glute hip-ups. For a full description of this exercise, see Chapter 4.

FIGURE 12-6:
Place your left foot close to your hips and pull your right knee to your chest (a) then raise your hips fully while pulling your right knee to your chest (b).

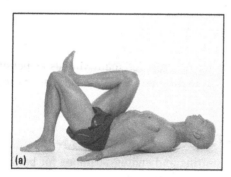 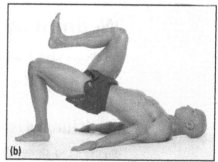

Photo by Jorge Alvarez, www.alvarezphoto.com

Windshield wipers

Figure 12-7 shows the starting and ending positions for windshield wipers. For a full description of this exercise, see Chapter 4.

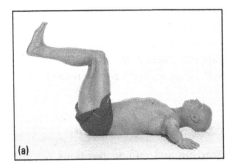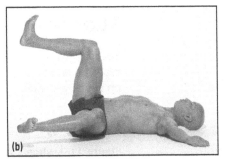

FIGURE 12-7: Place your arms at the T position and raise your legs over your hips (a) and then lower your left leg and right leg before reversing the movement (b).

Photo by Jorge Alvarez, www.alvarezphoto.com

Up and overs

Figure 12-8 shows the starting and ending positions for up and overs. For a full description of this exercise, see Chapter 4.

FIGURE 12-8: Make yourself long and straight with your arms at the T position (a) then pull your left knee to your chest while reaching up (b). Reset and repeat, except this time reach across your body.

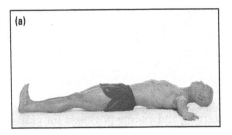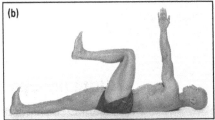

Photo by Jorge Alvarez, www.alvarezphoto.com

Wednesday

On Wednesday, it's time for AMRAPs (as many rounds as possible): Perform as many rounds as possible in 16 minutes. Alternate sides after each rep for single-sided exercises.

Back lunges (six reps)

Figure 12-9 shows the starting and ending positions for back lunges. For a full description of this exercise, see Chapter 7.

Tripod scissor kicks (eight reps)

Figure 12-10 shows the starting and ending positions for tripod scissor kicks. For a full description of this exercise, see Chapter 6.

FIGURE 12-9:
Stand tall with
your hands
behind your head
(a) and then take
a big backward
step while
maintaining an
upright torso (b).

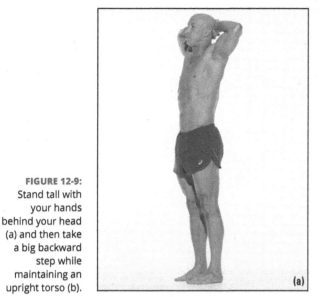

Photo by Jorge Alvarez, www.alvarezphoto.com

FIGURE 12-10:
Get into a
push-up position
with your feet
shoulder-width
apart (a) and then
bring your left leg
to your right leg
(b). Then reset to
the starting
position.

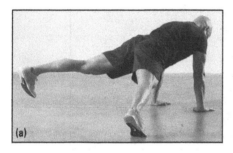
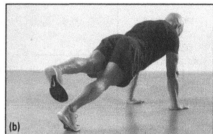

Photo by Jorge Alvarez, www.alvarezphoto.com

Romanian deadlifts (six reps)

Figure 12-11 shows the starting and ending positions for Romanian deadlifts. For a full description of this exercise, see Chapter 7.

Y-cuffs (eight reps)

Figure 12-12 shows the starting and ending positions for Y-cuffs. For a full description of this exercise, see Chapter 4.

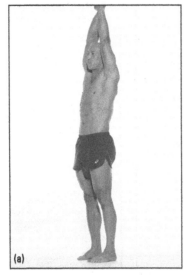
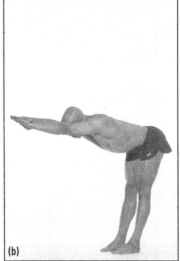

FIGURE 12-11: Stand with your feet hip-width apart and arms overhead (a) and then push your hips back and bend forward while keeping your legs and back straight (b).

Photo by Jorge Alvarez, www.alvarezphoto.com

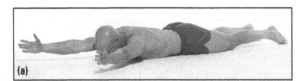
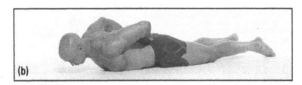

FIGURE 12-12: Lie on your stomach with your arms in the Y position (a), then place your hands on your lower back and lift your elbows (b).

Photo by Jorge Alvarez, www.alvarezphoto.com

Thursday

Thursday is the day for *crawling exercises*. Perform each exercise for a single set of six repetitions. For single-sided exercises, do all reps on your left side and then on your right side.

Dirty dogs

Figure 12-13 shows the starting and ending positions for dirty dogs. For a full description of this exercise, see Chapter 4.

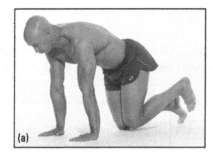
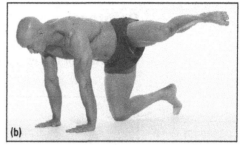

FIGURE 12-13: Get into a crawling position with your left knee slightly off the ground (a) and then raise your left knee as high as you can (b).

Photo by Jorge Alvarez, www.alvarezphoto.com

Hip circles

Figure 12-14 shows the starting and ending positions for hip circles. For a full description of this exercise, see Chapter 4.

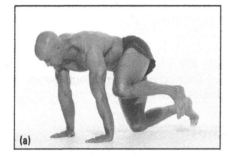
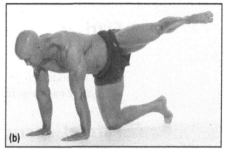

FIGURE 12-14: Get into a crawling position with your left knee slightly off the ground (a) and then make a giant circle with your knee going backward and forward (b).

Photo by Jorge Alvarez, www.alvarezphoto.com

Straight wide legs

Figure 12-15 shows the starting and ending positions for straight wide legs. For a full description of this exercise, see Chapter 4.

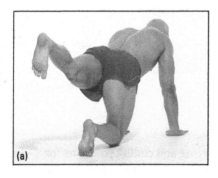
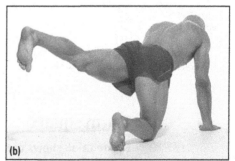

FIGURE 12-15: Get into a crawling position with your left leg fully extended (a) and then bring your left leg out to the left while keeping your left knee pointing straight down (b). Repeat on the right.

Photo by Jorge Alvarez, www.alvarezphoto.com

Pointers

Figure 12-16 shows the starting and ending positions for pointers. For a full description of this exercise, see Chapter 4.

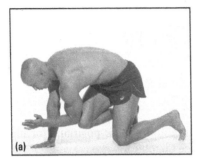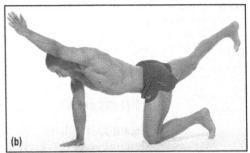

FIGURE 12-16: Bring your left elbow to your right knee (a) and then fully extend your left arm and right leg, raising them as high as you can (b).

Photo by Jorge Alvarez, www.alvarezphoto.com

Friday

Friday is your *circuit training* day. Perform each exercise for 40 seconds. Then rest for 20 seconds before doing the next movement. Complete three circuits. Alternate sides after each rep for single-sided exercises.

Parallel leg crunches

Figure 12-17 shows the starting and ending positions for parallel leg crunches. For a full description of this exercise, see Chapter 6.

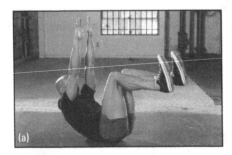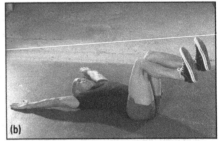

FIGURE 12-17: With your knees above your hips, reach up as high as you can with your arms (a) and then lie flat on your back while bringing your arms to the Y position (b).

Photo by Jorge Alvarez, www.alvarezphoto.com

T-arm squats

Figure 12-18 shows the starting and ending positions for T-arm squats crunches. For a full description of this exercise, see Chapter 7.

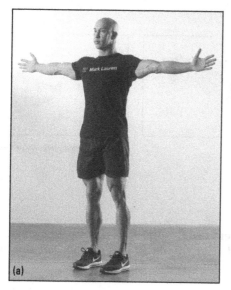

FIGURE 12-18: Stand with your arms at the T position and your feet hip-width apart (a) and then push your hips back and down while lifting your chest (b).

Photo by Jorge Alvarez, www.alvarezphoto.com

Starfish twists

Figure 12-19 shows the starting and ending positions for starfish twists. For a full description of this exercise, see Chapter 4.

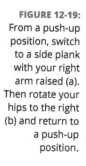

FIGURE 12-19: From a push-up position, switch to a side plank with your right arm raised (a). Then rotate your hips to the right (b) and return to a push-up position.

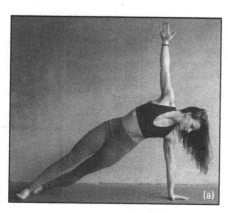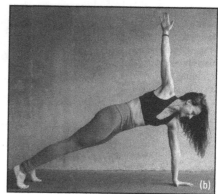

Photo by Jorge Alvarez, www.alvarezphoto.com

Skydivers arms at sides

Figure 12-20 shows the starting and ending positions for skydivers with your arms at the sides. For a full description of this exercise, see Chapter 6.

FIGURE 12-20:
Lie on your stomach with your arms at your sides and your feet together (a). While keeping your arms and legs off the ground, open and close your legs (b).

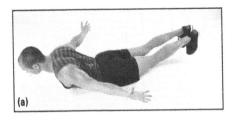 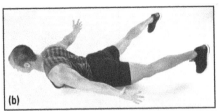

Photo by Jorge Alvarez, www.alvarezphoto.com

Saturday

Time for front lying exercises! Perform each exercise for a single set of six repetitions. For single-sided exercises, do all reps on your left side and then on your right side.

Hip twists

Figure 12-21 shows the starting and ending positions for hip twists. For a full description of this exercise, see Chapter 4.

FIGURE 12-21:
From a push-up position, roll your heels to the right (a), and then roll your heels to the left while keeping your hips centered (b).

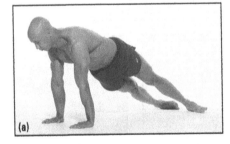 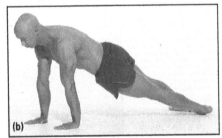

Photo by Jorge Alvarez, www.alvarezphoto.com

Moose antlers

Figure 12-22 shows the starting and ending positions for moose antlers. For a full description of this exercise, see Chapter 4.

Twists and reaches

Figure 12-23 shows the starting and ending positions for twists and reaches. For a full description of this exercise, see Chapter 4.

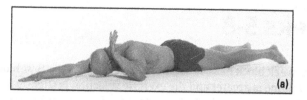

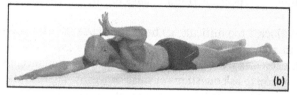

FIGURE 12-22: Reach your right arm past your head and place your left thumb on the back of your head (a). Then press your right hand into the ground and lift your left elbow as high as you can (b).

Photo by Jorge Alvarez, www.alvarezphoto.com

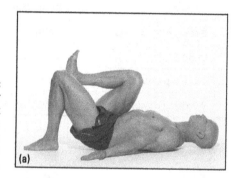 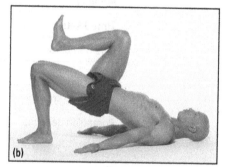

FIGURE 12-23: Reach under your body to the right with your left arm (a) and then reach up as high as you can (b).

Photo by Jorge Alvarez, www.alvarezphoto.com

Y-cuffs

Figure 12-24 shows the starting and ending positions for Y-cuffs. For a full description of this exercise, see Chapter 4.

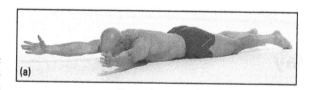

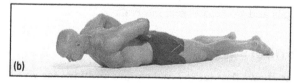

FIGURE 12-24: Reach your arms to the Y position with your thumbs up (a) and then place your hands on your lower back and raise your elbows (b).

Photo by Jorge Alvarez, www.alvarezphoto.com

Block 2: Weeks 5-8

This four-week block has the same workout types as the first block. However, the training volume is greater and the exercise selection is slightly more difficult. Just like with Block 1, repeat the training days for four weeks before moving on.

TIP

If you find Block 2 too difficult, go back and repeat Block 1 before trying again. If you want to stay on Block 2 but find some of the exercises too difficult, replace them with exercises from Block 1. For personalized guidance, use the chat tool at marklauren.com to ask questions or raise concerns. There is also a very active and supportive community that's free to join at community.marklauren.com.

Monday	Tuesday	Wednesday
Timed Sets	**Back Lying Exercises**	**AMRAP**
Dive bombers	Dead bugs	Glute hip-ups
T-arm squats	Glute hip-ups	Deep squats
Parallel leg crunches	Windshield wipers	Starfish twists
Romanian deadlifts	Up and overs	Back lunges

Thursday	Friday	Saturday
Crawling Exercises	**Circuit Training**	**Front Lying Exercises**
Dirty dogs	Mountain climbers	Hip twists
Hip circles	Side lunges	Moose antlers
Straight wide legs	Scorpion kicks	Twists and reaches
Pointers	Skydivers arms at T	Y-cuffs

Monday

Monday means timed sets. Perform each exercise for four sets using 35-second work intervals and 35-second rest intervals.

Dive bombers

Figure 12-25 shows the starting and ending positions for dive bombers. For a full description of this exercise, see Chapter 8.

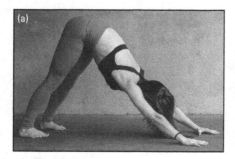
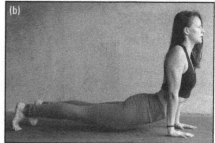

FIGURE 12-25:
From a push-up position, push your hips up and your chest down (a) then lower your hips to the ground and lift your chest (b).

T-arm squats

Figure 12-26 shows the starting and ending positions for T-arm squats. For a full description of this exercise, see Chapter 7.

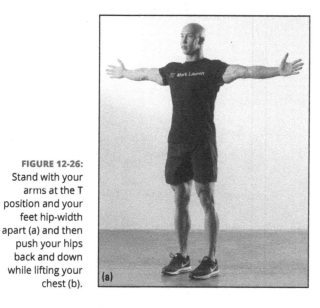
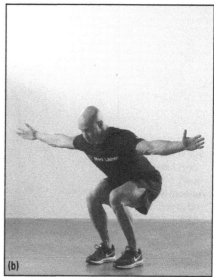

FIGURE 12-26:
Stand with your arms at the T position and your feet hip-width apart (a) and then push your hips back and down while lifting your chest (b).

Parallel leg crunches

Figure 12-27 shows the starting and ending positions for parallel leg crunches. For a full description of this exercise, see Chapter 6.

FIGURE 12-27:
With your knees
above your hips,
reach up as high
as you can with
your arms (a) and
then lie flat on
your back while
bringing your
arms to the Y
position (b).

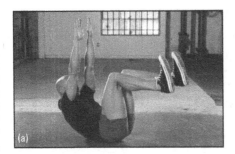 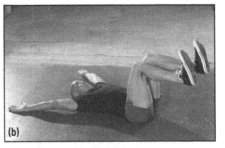

Photo by Jorge Alvarez, www.alvarezphoto.com

Romanian deadlifts

Figure 12-28 shows the starting and ending positions for Romanian deadlifts. For a full description of this exercise, see Chapter 7.

FIGURE 12-28:
Stand with your
feet hip-width
apart and arms
overhead (a) then
push your hips
back and bend
forward while
keeping your legs
and back straight.

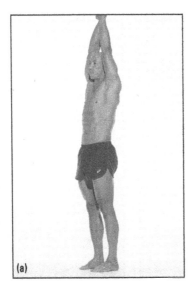 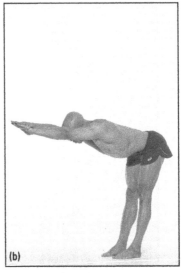

Photo by Jorge Alvarez, www.alvarezphoto.com

Tuesday

Tuesday means back lying exercises. Perform each exercise for a single set of eight repetitions. For single-sided exercises, do all reps on your left side and then on your right side.

Dead bugs

Figure 12-29 shows the starting and ending positions for dead bugs. For a full description of this exercise, see Chapter 4.

FIGURE 12-29: Lie on your back with your knees directly over your hips (a) and then extend your left leg fully while pressing your lower back into the ground (b).

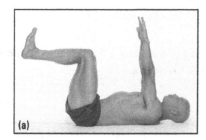 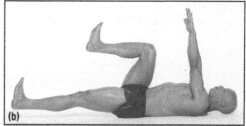

Photo by Jorge Alvarez, www.alvarezphoto.com

Glute hip-ups

Figure 12-30 shows the starting and ending positions for glute hip-ups. For a full description of this exercise, see Chapter 4.

FIGURE 12-30: Place your left foot close to your hips and pull your right knee to your chest (a), then raise your hips fully while pulling your right knee to your chest (b).

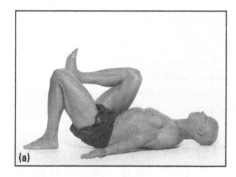 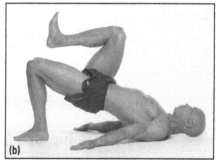

Photo by Jorge Alvarez, www.alvarezphoto.com

Windshield wipers

Figure 12-31 shows the starting and ending positions for windshield wipers. For a full description of this exercise, see Chapter 4.

FIGURE 12-31: Place your arms at the T position and raise your legs over your hips (a). Then alternately lower your left leg and right leg in turn (b).

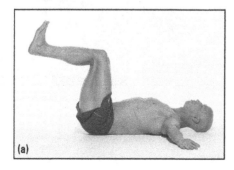 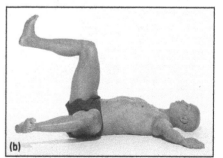

Photo by Jorge Alvarez, www.alvarezphoto.com

Up and overs

Figure 12-32 shows the starting and ending positions for up and overs. For a full description of this exercise, see Chapter 4.

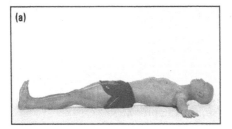 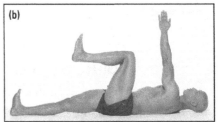

Photo by Jorge Alvarez, www.alvarezphoto.com

Wednesday

Wednesday means it's time for AMRAPs (as many rounds as possible). Perform as many rounds as you can in 18 minutes using good form. Alternate sides after each rep for single-sided exercises.

Glute hip-ups (six reps each side)

Figure 12-33 shows the starting and ending positions for parallel leg bridges. For a full description of this exercise, see Chapter 4.

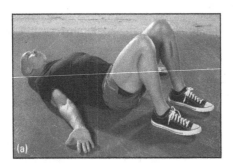 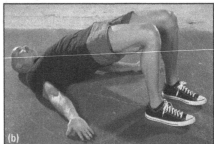

Photo by Jorge Alvarez, www.alvarezphoto.com

Deep squats (four reps)

Figure 12-34 shows the starting and ending positions for deep squats. For a full description of this exercise, see Chapter 10.

FIGURE 12-34:
Start in a push-up position with your feet hip-width apart (a) and then walk your hips back and get into the bottom of a squat (b). Stand up tall.

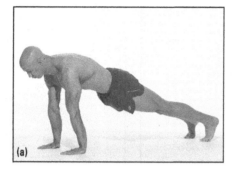 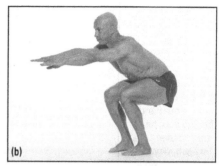

Photo by Jorge Alvarez, www.alvarezphoto.com

Starfish twists (four reps)

Figure 12-35 shows the starting and ending positions for starfish twists. For a full description of this exercise, see Chapter 10.

FIGURE 12-35:
From a push-up position, switch to a side plank with your right arm raised (a) and then rotate your hips to the right and return to a push-up position (b).

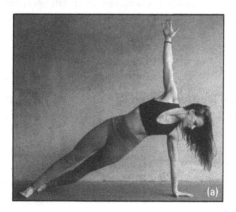 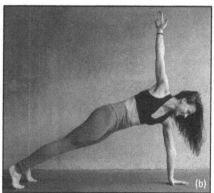

Photo by Jorge Alvarez, www.alvarezphoto.com

Back lunges (six reps)

Figure 12-36 shows the starting and ending positions for back lunges. For a full description of this exercise, see Chapter 7.

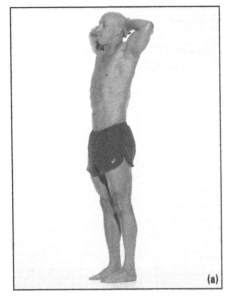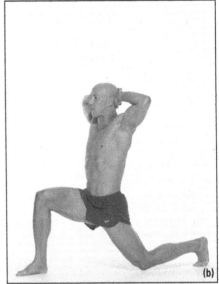

FIGURE 12-36: Stand tall with your hands behind your head (a) and then take a big backwards step while maintaining an upright torso (b).

Photo by Jorge Alvarez, www.alvarezphoto.com

Thursday

Get ready! Thursday means crawling exercises. Perform each exercise for a single set of eight repetitions. For single-sided exercises, do all reps on your left side and then on your right side.

Dirty dogs

Figure 12-37 shows the starting and ending positions for dirty dogs. For a full description of this exercise, see Chapter 4.

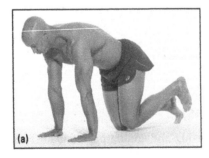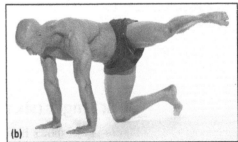

FIGURE 12-37: Get into a crawling position with your left knee slightly off the ground (a) and then raise your left knee as high as you can (b).

Photo by Jorge Alvarez, www.alvarezphoto.com

Hip circles

Figure 12-38 shows the starting and ending positions for hip circles. For a full description of this exercise, see Chapter 4.

FIGURE 12-38:
Get into a crawling position with your left knee slightly off the ground (a) and then make a giant circle with your knee going backward and forward (b).

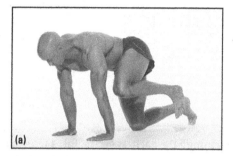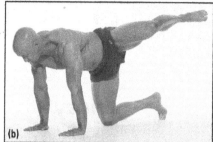

Photo by Jorge Alvarez, www.alvarezphoto.com

Straight wide legs

Figure 12-39 shows the starting and ending positions for straight wide legs. For a full description of this exercise, see Chapter 4.

FIGURE 12-39:
Get into a crawling position with your left leg fully extended (a) and then bring your left leg out to your left while keeping your left knee pointing straight down (b).

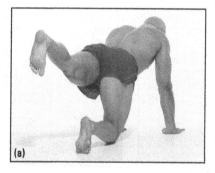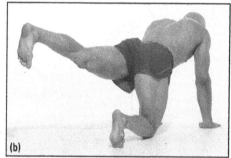

Photo by Jorge Alvarez, www.alvarezphoto.com

Pointers

Figure 12-40 shows the starting and ending positions for pointers. For a full description of this exercise, see Chapter 4.

FIGURE 12-40:
Bring your left
elbow to your
right knee (a) and
then fully extend
your left arm and
right leg, raising
them as high as
you can (b).

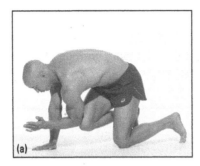 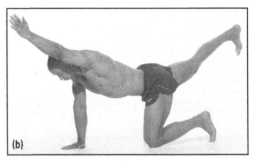

Photo by Jorge Alvarez, www.alvarezphoto.com

Friday

Friday equals circuit training! Do each exercise for 35 seconds. Then rest for 20 seconds before moving on to the next exercise. Complete four circuits. Alternate sides after each rep for single-sided exercises.

Mountain climbers

Figure 12-41 shows the starting and ending positions for mountain climbers. For a full description of this exercise, see Chapter 6.

FIGURE 12-41:
Get into the
starting position
of a push-up (a).
Then alternate
bringing your
knees to your
elbows, as if
you're running in
place while
maintaining a
straight push-up
position (b).

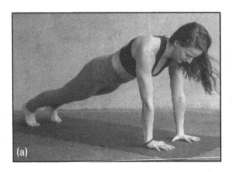 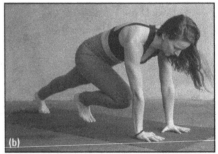

Photo by Jorge Alvarez, www.alvarezphoto.com

Side lunges

Figure 12-42 shows the starting and ending positions for side lunges. For a full description of this exercise, see Chapter 7.

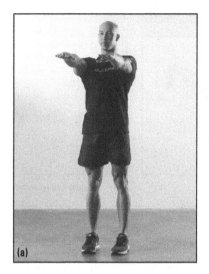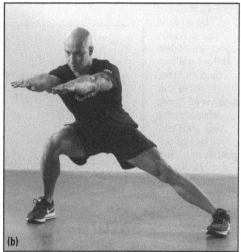

FIGURE 12-42:
Stand tall with your arms extended to the front (a). Then take a giant step to the side, push your hips back and lift your chest up (b).

Photo by Jorge Alvarez, www.alvarezphoto.com

Scorpion kicks

Figure 12-43 shows the starting and ending positions for scorpion kicks. For a full description of this exercise, see Chapter 6.

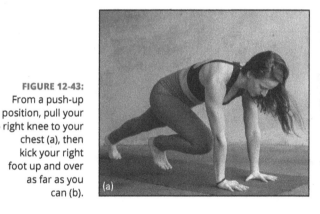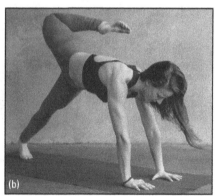

FIGURE 12-43:
From a push-up position, pull your right knee to your chest (a), then kick your right foot up and over as far as you can (b).

Photo by Jorge Alvarez, www.alvarezphoto.com

Skydivers arms at T

Figure 12-44 shows the starting and ending positions for skydiver arms at T. For a full description of this exercise, see Chapter 6.

FIGURE 12-44:
Lie on your stomach with your arms lifted at the T position and your feet lifted and together (a). Then, while keeping your arms and legs off the ground, open and close your legs (b).

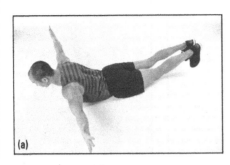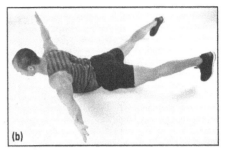

Photo by Jorge Alvarez, www.alvarezphoto.com

Saturday

Saturday calls for front lying exercises. Perform each exercise for a single set of six repetitions. For single-sided exercises, do all reps on your left side and then on your right side.

Hip twists

Figure 12-45 shows the starting and ending positions for hip twists. For a full description of this exercise, see Chapter 4.

FIGURE 12-45:
From a push-up position, roll your heels to the right (a) and then roll your heels to the left while keeping your hips centered (b).

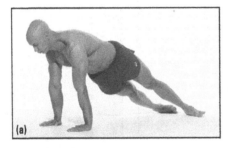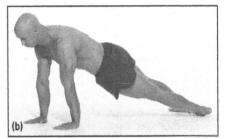

Photo by Jorge Alvarez, www.alvarezphoto.com

Moose antlers

Figure 12-46 shows the starting and ending positions for moose antlers. For a full description of this exercise, see Chapter 4.

Twists and reaches

Figure 12-47 shows the starting and ending positions for twists and reaches. For a full description of this exercise, see Chapter 4.

FIGURE 12-46:
Reach your right arm past your head and place your left thumb on the back of your head (a). Then press your right hand into the ground and lift your left elbow as high as you can (b).

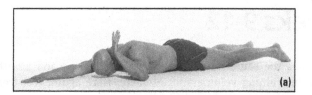
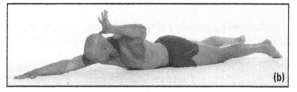

Photo by Jorge Alvarez, www.alvarezphoto.com

FIGURE 12-47:
Reach under your body to the right with your left arm (a) and then reach up as high as you can (b).

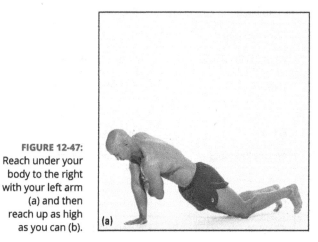
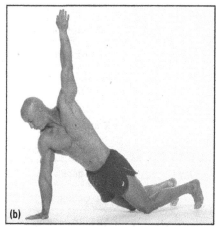

Photo by Jorge Alvarez, www.alvarezphoto.com

Y-cuffs

Figure 12-48 shows the starting and ending positions for Y-cuffs. For a full description of this exercise, see Chapter 4.

FIGURE 12-48:
Reach your arms to the Y position with your thumbs up (a) and then place your hands on your lower back and raise your elbows (b).

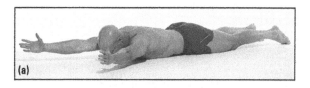
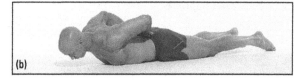

Photo by Jorge Alvarez, www.alvarezphoto.com

Block 3: Weeks 9-12

Block 3 has the same training structure as Blocks 1 and 2 with another slight increase in training volume and intensity. Here again, feel free to replace any movements that you find too difficult.

You repeat the following training days for four weeks before moving on to the last week of this program, which is the active recovery week.

Monday	Tuesday	Wednesday
Timed Sets	**Back Lying Exercises**	**AMRAP**
V-ups	Dead bugs	DF glides
Squat thrusts	Glute hip-ups	Saxon lunges
Skydivers arms at Y	Windshield wipers	Starfish hip drops
Kickouts	Up and overs	Deadlifts to squats

Thursday	Friday	Saturday
Crawling Exercises	**Circuit Training**	**Front Lying Exercises**
Dirty dogs	Reaching bodyrocks	Hip twists
Hip circles	Saxon lunges	Moose antlers
Straight wide legs	Kickouts	Twists and reaches
Pointers	Squats to deadlifts	Y-cuffs

Monday

Monday means timed sets. Perform each exercise for five sets using 30-second work intervals and 30-second rest intervals. Alternate sides after each rep for single-sided exercises.

V-ups

Figure 12-49 shows the starting and ending positions for V-ups. For a full description of this exercise, see Chapter 6.

FIGURE 12-49:
Make yourself
long with your
arms and legs
slightly off the
ground (a) and
then bring your
chest to your
knees, while
keeping your
back straight (b).

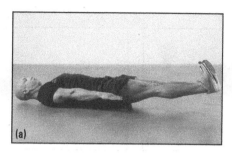 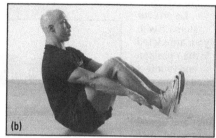

Photo by Jorge Alvarez, www.alvarezphoto.com

Squat thrusts

Figure 12-50 shows the starting and ending positions for squat thrusts. For a full description of this exercise, see Chapter 7.

FIGURE 12-50:
Get into the
bottom of a squat
with your arms in
front of you (a)
and then place
your hands on
the ground and
kick your legs
back into a
plank (b).

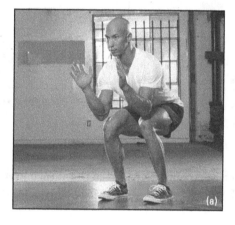 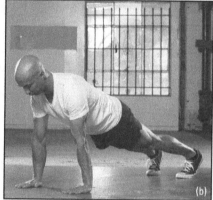

Photo by Jorge Alvarez, www.alvarezphoto.com

Skydivers arms at Y

Figure 12-51 shows the starting and ending positions for skydivers arms at Y. For a full description of this exercise, see Chapter 6.

Kickouts

Figure 12-52 shows the starting and ending positions for kickouts. For a full description of this exercise, see Chapter 10.

FIGURE 12-51: Lie on your stomach with your arms lifted in the Y position and your feet lifted together (a) then, while keeping your arms and legs off the ground, open and close your legs (b).

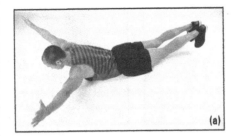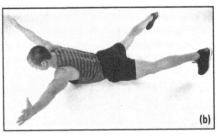

Photo by Jorge Alvarez, www.alvarezphoto.com

FIGURE 12-52: Get into a quadruped position with your knees off the ground (a) then rotate to the right and perform a kickout with your left leg (b). Repeat with the opposite leg.

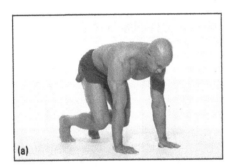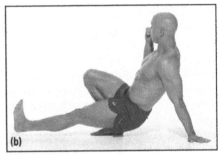

Photo by Jorge Alvarez, www.alvarezphoto.com

Tuesday

It's Tuesday — time for back lying exercises! Perform each exercise for a single set of ten repetitions. For single-sided exercises, do all reps on your left side and then on your right side.

Dead bugs

Figure 12-53 shows the starting and ending positions for dead bugs. For a full description of this exercise, see Chapter 4.

FIGURE 12-53: Lie on your back with your knees directly over your hips (a) and then extend your left leg fully while pressing your lower back into the ground (b).

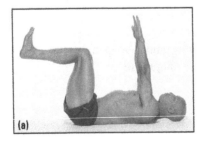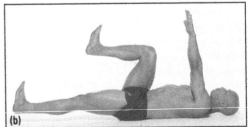

Photo by Jorge Alvarez, www.alvarezphoto.com

Glute hip-ups

Figure 12-54 shows the starting and ending positions for glute hip-ups. For a full description of this exercise, see Chapter 4.

FIGURE 12-54: Place your left foot close to your hips and pull your right knee to your chest (a) and then raise your hips fully while pulling your right knee to your chest (b).

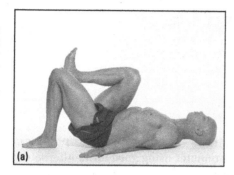
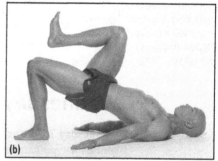

Photo by Jorge Alvarez, www.alvarezphoto.com

Windshield wipers

Figure 12-55 shows the starting and ending positions for windshield wipers. For a full description of this exercise, see Chapter 4.

FIGURE 12-55: Place your arms at the T position and raise your legs over your hips (a). Then lower your left leg and right leg in alternating movements (b).

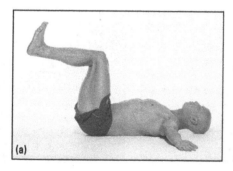
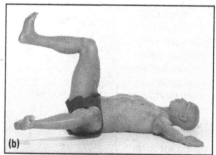

Photo by Jorge Alvarez, www.alvarezphoto.com

Up and overs

Figure 12-56 shows the starting and ending positions for up and overs. For a full description of this exercise, see Chapter 4.

FIGURE 12-56:
Make yourself
long and straight
with your arms at
the T position (a).
Then pull your
left knee to your
chest while
reaching up with
your left arm (b).
Repeat and reach
across your body.

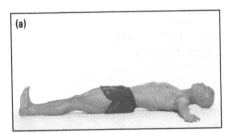 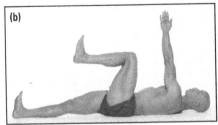

Photo by Jorge Alvarez, www.alvarezphoto.com

Wednesday

Wednesday calls for AMRAPs (as many rounds as possible). Perform as many rounds as you can in 20 minutes using good form. Alternate sides after each rep for single-sided exercises.

DF glides (five reps)

Figure 12-57 shows the starting and ending positions for DF glides. For a full description of this exercise, see Chapter 8.

FIGURE 12-57:
Get into the
bottom of a
push-up position
with your hands
under your
shoulders (a).
Then push your
hips up and back
as far as possible
while pushing
your chest down
toward your
hands (b).

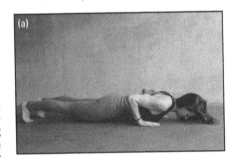 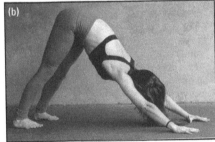

Photo by Jorge Alvarez, www.alvarezphoto.com

Saxon lunges (four reps)

Figure 12-58 shows the starting and ending positions for Saxon lunges. For a full description of this exercise, see Chapter 7.

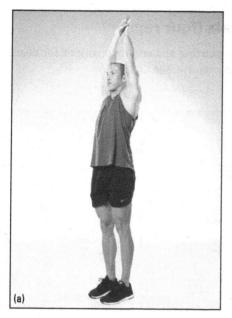
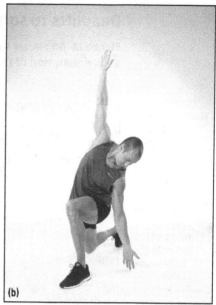

FIGURE 12-58:
Stand with your
arms overhead at
the streamline
position (a). After
stepping into a
back lunge, reach
down on the side
of the lead leg (b).

(a)

(b)

Photo by Jorge Alvarez, www.alvarezphoto.com

Starfish hip drops (four reps)

Figure 12-59 shows the starting and ending positions for starfish hip drops. For a
full description of this exercise, see Chapter 10.

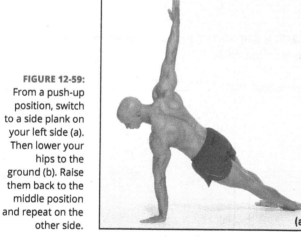
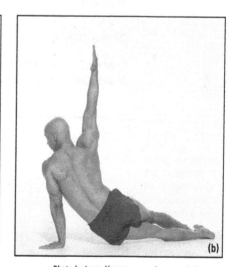

FIGURE 12-59:
From a push-up
position, switch
to a side plank on
your left side (a).
Then lower your
hips to the
ground (b). Raise
them back to the
middle position
and repeat on the
other side.

(a)

(b)

Photo by Jorge Alvarez, www.alvarezphoto.com

Deadlifts to squats (four reps)

Figure 12-60 shows the starting and ending positions for deadlifts to squats. For a full description of this exercise, see Chapter 7.

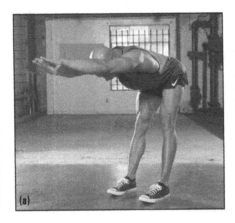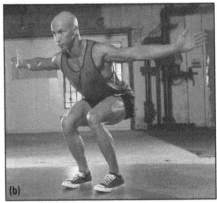

FIGURE 12-60: From a standing position, bend forward until you're in the bottom of a Romanian deadlift (a). Switch to the bottom of a T-arm squat (b). Return to the bottom of a Romanian deadlift and then stand up.

Photo by Jorge Alvarez, www.alvarezphoto.com

Thursday

You do crawling exercises on Tuesday. Perform each exercise for a single set of ten repetitions. For single-sided exercises, do all reps on your left side and then on your right side.

Dirty dogs

Figure 12-61 shows the starting and ending positions for dirty dogs. For a full description of this exercise, see Chapter 4.

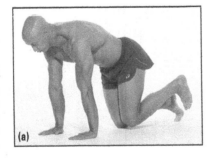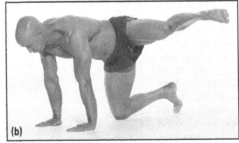

FIGURE 12-61: Get into a crawling position with your left knee slightly off the ground (a) and then raise your left knee as high as you can (b).

Photo by Jorge Alvarez, www.alvarezphoto.com

Hip circles

Figure 12-62 shows the starting and ending positions for hip circles. For a full description of this exercise, see Chapter 4.

FIGURE 12-62:
Get into a crawling position with your left knee slightly off the ground (a), then make a giant circle with your knee going backward and forward (b).

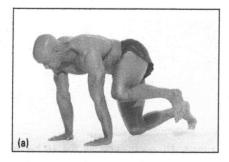 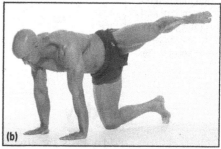

Photo by Jorge Alvarez, www.alvarezphoto.com

Straight wide legs

Figure 12-63 shows the starting and ending positions for straight wide legs. For a full description of this exercise, see Chapter 4.

FIGURE 12-63:
Get into a crawling position with your left leg fully extended (a) and then bring your left leg out to your left while keeping your left knee pointing straight down (b).

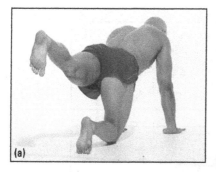 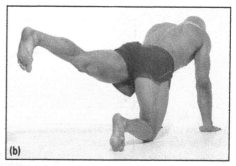

Photo by Jorge Alvarez, www.alvarezphoto.com

Pointers

Figure 12-64 shows the starting and ending positions for pointers. For a full description of this exercise, see Chapter 4.

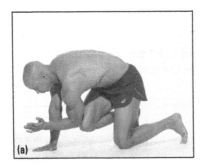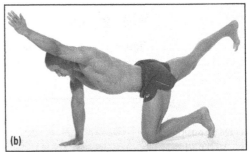

FIGURE 12-64: Bring your left elbow to your right knee (a) and then fully extend your left arm and right leg, raising them as high as you can (b).

Photo by Jorge Alvarez, www.alvarezphoto.com

Friday

Friday calls for circuit training. Do each exercise for 30 seconds. Then rest for 20 seconds before moving on to the next exercise. Complete five circuits. Alternate sides after each rep for single-sided exercises.

Reaching bodyrocks

Figure 12-65 shows the starting and ending positions for reaching bodyrocks. For a full description of this exercise, see Chapter 6.

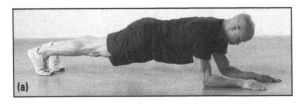
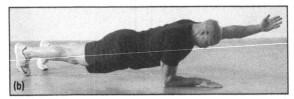

FIGURE 12-65: Get into a straight planking position on your forearms (a) and then rock forward and backward as far you can (b).

Photo by Jorge Alvarez, www.alvarezphoto.com

Saxon lunges

Figure 12-66 shows the starting and ending positions for Saxon lunges. For a full description of this exercise, see Chapter 7.

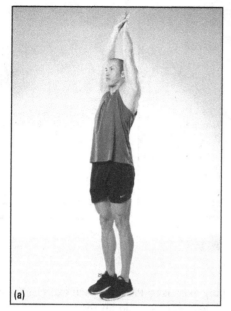
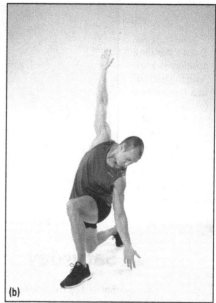

Photo by Jorge Alvarez, www.alvarezphoto.com

FIGURE 12-66: Stand with your arms overhead at the Streamline position (a). After stepping into a back lunge, reach down on the side of the lead leg (b).

Kickouts

Figure 12-67 shows the starting and ending positions for kickouts. For a full description of this exercise, see Chapter 10.

FIGURE 12-67: Get into a quadruped position with your knees off the ground (a) and then rotate to the right and perform a kickout with your left leg (b). Repeat with the other leg.

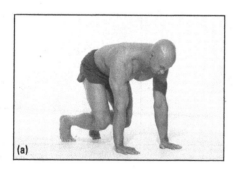
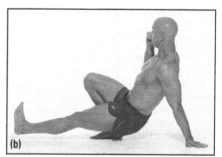

Photo by Jorge Alvarez, www.alvarezphoto.com

Squats to deadlifts

Figure 12-68 shows the starting and ending positions for squats to deadlifts. For a full description of this exercise, see Chapter 7.

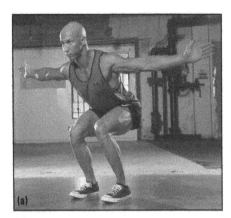
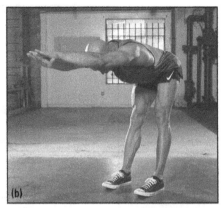

FIGURE 12-68: From a standing position, sit back into the bottom of a T-arm squat (a). Switch to the bottom of a Romanian deadlift (b). Return to the bottom of a T-arm squat and then stand up.

Photo by Jorge Alvarez, www.alvarezphoto.com

Saturday

Saturday means front lying exercises. Perform each exercise for a single set of ten repetitions. For single-sided exercises, do all reps on your left side and then on your right side.

Hip twists

Figure 12-69 shows the starting and ending positions for hip twists. For a full description of this exercise, see Chapter 4.

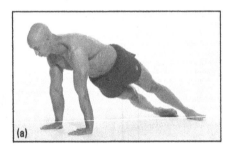
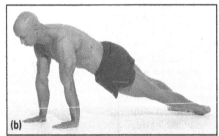

FIGURE 12-69: From a push-up position, roll your heels to the right (a) and then roll your heels to the left while keeping your hips centered (b).

Photo by Jorge Alvarez, www.alvarezphoto.com

Moose antlers

Figure 12-70 shows the starting and ending positions for moose antlers. For a full description of this exercise, see Chapter 4.

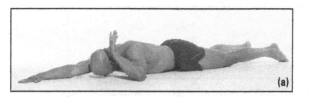

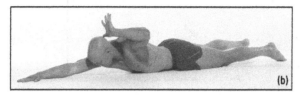

FIGURE 12-70:
Reach your right arm past your head and place your left thumb on the back of your head (a). Then press your right hand into the ground and lift your left elbow as high as you can (b).

Photo by Jorge Alvarez, www.alvarezphoto.com

Twists and reaches

Figure 12-71 shows the starting and ending positions for twists and reaches. For a full description of this exercise, see Chapter 4.

FIGURE 12-71:
Reach under your body to the right with your left arm (a) and then reach up as high as you can (b).

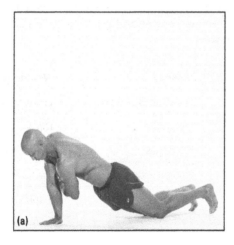

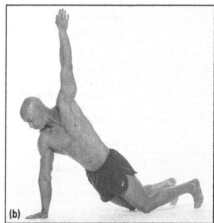

Photo by Jorge Alvarez, www.alvarezphoto.com

Y-cuffs

Figure 12-72 shows the starting and ending positions for Y-cuffs. For a full description of this exercise, see Chapter 4.

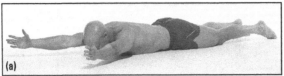

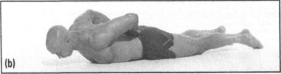

FIGURE 12-72: Reach your arms to the Y position with your thumbs up (a) and then place your hands on your lower back and raise your elbows (b).

Photo by Jorge Alvarez, www.alvarezphoto.com

The Active Recovery Week

Congratulations — this is your final week of the program! The purpose of this week's training is to ensure full recovery and preparedness before repeating this program or moving on to your next training routine. Week 13 is made up of light workouts using only floor exercises. These exercises will help improve your mobility while allowing you to recover and get back to full strength. Here is an overview of the training week.

Monday	Tuesday	Wednesday
Back Lying Exercises	**Crawling Exercises**	**Front Lying Exercises**
Dead bugs	Dirty dogs	Hip twists
Glute hip-ups	Hip circles	Moose antlers
Windshield wipers	Straight wide legs	Twists and reaches
Up and overs	Pointers	Y-cuffs

Thursday	Friday	Saturday
Back Lying Exercises	**Crawling Exercises**	**Front Lying Exercises**
Dead bugs	Dirty dogs	Hip twists
Glute hip-ups	Hip circles	Moose antlers
Windshield wipers	Straight wide legs	Twists and reaches
Up and overs	Pointers	Y-cuffs

Monday

Monday means back lying exercises. Perform each exercise for a single set of six repetitions. For single-sided exercises, do all reps on your left side and then on your right side. You can find the full exercise descriptions for all these movements in Chapter 4.

Dead bugs

Figure 12-73 shows the starting and ending positions for dead bugs.

FIGURE 12-73: Lie on your back with your knees directly over your hips (a) and then extend your left leg fully while pressing your lower back into the ground (b).

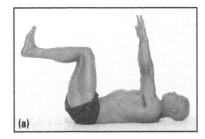 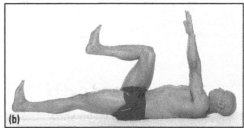

Photo by Jorge Alvarez, www.alvarezphoto.com

Glute hip-ups

Figure 12-74 shows the starting and ending positions for glute hip-ups.

FIGURE 12-74: Place your left foot close to your hips and pull your right knee to your chest (a), then raise your hips fully while pulling the right knee to your chest (b).

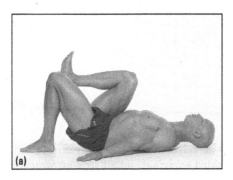 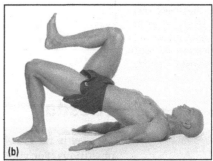

Photo by Jorge Alvarez, www.alvarezphoto.com

Windshield wipers

Figure 12-75 shows the starting and ending positions for windshield wipers.

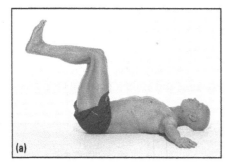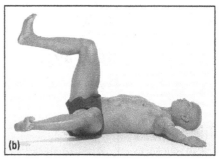

FIGURE 12-75: Place your arms at the T position and raise your legs over your hips (a). Lower your left leg then right leg, reversing the movement (b).

Photo by Jorge Alvarez, www.alvarezphoto.com

Up and overs

Figure 12-76 shows the starting and ending positions for up and overs.

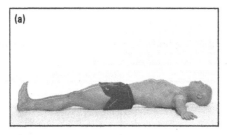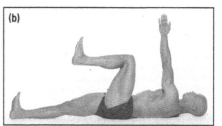

FIGURE 12-76: Make yourself long and straight with your arms at the T position (a) and then pull your left knee to your chest while reaching up with your left arm (b). Repeat and reach across your body.

Photo by Jorge Alvarez, www.alvarezphoto.com

Tuesday

Tuesday is for crawling exercises. Perform each exercise for a single set of six repetitions. For single-sided exercises, do all reps on your left side and then on your right side.

Dirty dogs

Figure 12-77 shows the starting and ending positions for dirty dogs.

FIGURE 12-77:
Get into a
crawling position
with your left
knee slightly off
the ground (a)
and raise your
left knee as high
as you can (b).

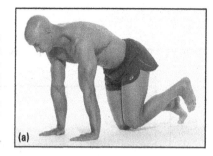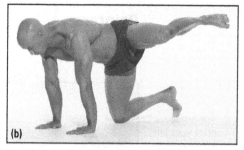

Photo by Jorge Alvarez, www.alvarezphoto.com

Hip circles

Figure 12-78 shows the starting and ending positions for hip circles.

FIGURE 12-78:
Get into a
crawling position
with your left
knee slightly off
the ground (a)
and then make a
giant circle with
your knee going
backward and
forward (b).

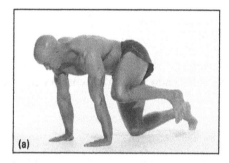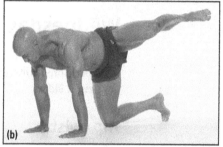

Photo by Jorge Alvarez, www.alvarezphoto.com

Straight wide legs

Figure 12-79 shows the starting and ending positions for straight wide legs.

FIGURE 12-79:
Get into a
crawling position
with your left leg
fully extended (a).
Bring your left leg
out to your left
while keeping
your left knee
pointing straight
down (b).

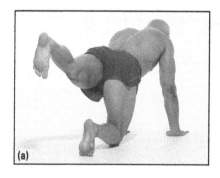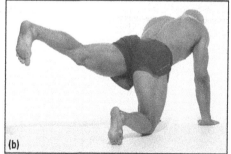

Photo by Jorge Alvarez, www.alvarezphoto.com

Pointers

Figure 12-80 shows the starting and ending positions for pointers.

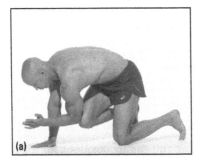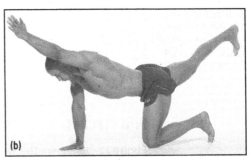

Photo by Jorge Alvarez, www.alvarezphoto.com

Wednesday

Wednesday means front lying exercises. Perform each exercise for a single set of six repetitions. For single-sided exercises, do all reps on your left side and then on your right side.

Hip twists

Figure 12-81 shows the starting and ending positions for hip twists.

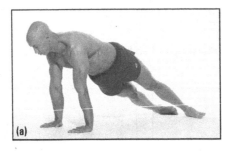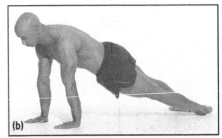

Photo by Jorge Alvarez, www.alvarezphoto.com

Moose antlers

Figure 12-82 shows the starting and ending positions for moose antlers.

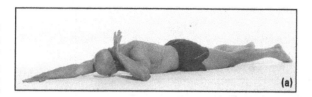

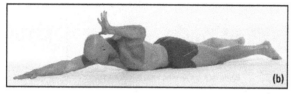

FIGURE 12-82:
Reach the right arm past your head and place your left thumb on the back of your head (a). Then press your right hand into the ground and lift your left elbow as high as you can (b).

Photo by Jorge Alvarez, www.alvarezphoto.com

Twists and reaches

Figure 12-83 shows the starting and ending positions for twists and reaches.

FIGURE 12-83:
Reach under your body to the right with your left arm (a) and reach up as high as you can (b).

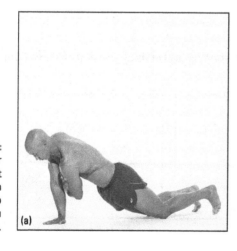

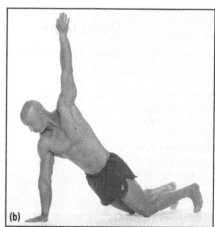

Photo by Jorge Alvarez, www.alvarezphoto.com

Y-cuffs

Figure 12-84 shows the starting and ending positions for Y-cuffs.

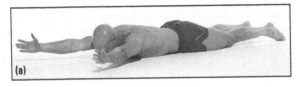

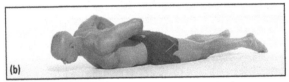

FIGURE 12-84: Reach your arms to the Y position with your thumbs up (a), then place your hands on your lower back and raise your elbows (b).

Photo by Jorge Alvarez, www.alvarezphoto.com

Thursday

Thursday means back lying exercises. Perform each exercise for a single set of six repetitions. For single-sided exercises, do all reps on your left side and then on your right side.

Dead bugs

Figure 12-85 shows the starting and ending positions for dead bugs.

FIGURE 12-85: Lie on your back with your knees directly over your hips (a) and then extend your left leg fully while pressing your lower back into the ground (b).

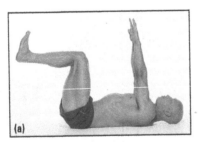 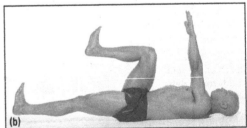

Photo by Jorge Alvarez, www.alvarezphoto.com

Glute hip-ups

Figure 12-86 shows the starting and ending positions for glute hip-ups.

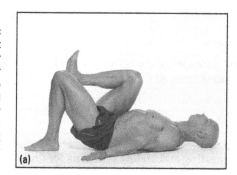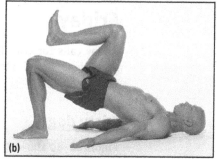

FIGURE 12-86: Place your left foot close to your hips and pull your right knee to your chest (a) and then raise your hips fully while pulling the right knee to your chest (b).

Photo by Jorge Alvarez, www.alvarezphoto.com

Windshield wipers

Figure 12-87 shows the starting and ending positions for windshield wipers.

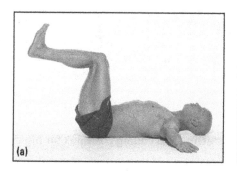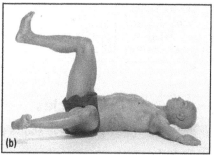

FIGURE 12-87: Place your arms at the T position and raise your legs over your hips (a). Then lower your left leg and right leg, alternating the movement (b).

Photo by Jorge Alvarez, www.alvarezphoto.com

Up and overs

Figure 12-88 shows the starting and ending positions for up and overs.

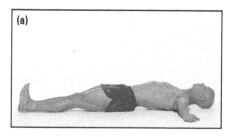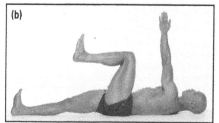

FIGURE 12-88: Make yourself long and straight with your arms at the T position (a). Then pull your left knee to your chest while reaching up with your left arm (b). Repeat and reach across your body.

Photo by Jorge Alvarez, www.alvarezphoto.com

Friday

Friday calls for crawling exercises. Perform each exercise for a single set of ten repetitions. For single-sided exercises, do all reps on your left side and then on your right side.

Dirty dogs

Figure 12-89 shows the starting and ending positions for dirty dogs.

FIGURE 12-89: Get into a crawling position with your left knee slightly off the ground (a) and then raise your left knee as high as you can (b).

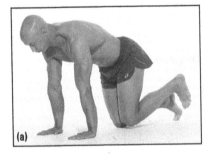 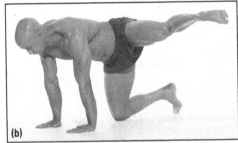

Photo by Jorge Alvarez, www.alvarezphoto.com

Hip circles

Figure 12-90 shows the starting and ending positions for hip circles.

FIGURE 12-90: Get into a crawling position with your left knee slightly off the ground (a) and then make a giant circle with your knee going backward and forward (b).

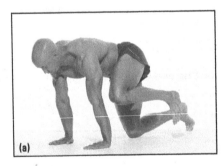 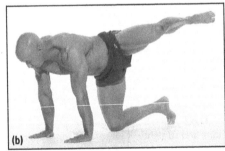

Photo by Jorge Alvarez, www.alvarezphoto.com

Straight wide legs

Figure 12-91 shows the starting and ending positions for straight wide legs.

FIGURE 12-91:
Get into a
crawling position
with your left leg
fully extended (a)
and then bring
your left leg out
to your left while
keeping your left
knee pointing
straight down (b).

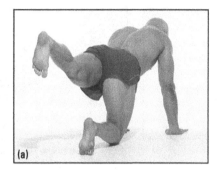 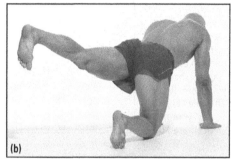

Photo by Jorge Alvarez, www.alvarezphoto.com

Pointers

Figure 12-92 shows the starting and ending positions for pointers.

FIGURE 12-92:
Bring your left
elbow to your
right knee (a).
Then fully extend
your left arm and
right leg, raising
them as high as
you can (b).

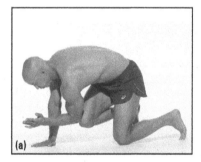 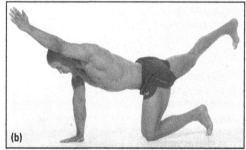

Photo by Jorge Alvarez, www.alvarezphoto.com

Saturday

Saturday means front lying exercises. Perform each exercise for a single set of six repetitions. For single-sided exercises, do all reps on your left side and then on your right side.

Hip twists

Figure 12-93 shows the starting and ending positions for hip twists.

FIGURE 12-93:
From a push-up position, roll your heels to the right (a) and then roll your heels to the left while keeping your hips centered (b).

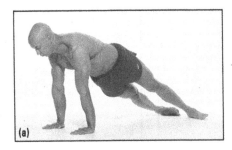 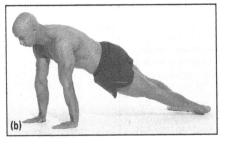

Photo by Jorge Alvarez, www.alvarezphoto.com

Moose antlers

Figure 12-94 shows the starting and ending positions for moose antlers.

FIGURE 12-94:
Reach your right arm past your head and place your left thumb on the back of your head (a). Then press your right hand into the ground and lift your left elbow as high as you can (b).

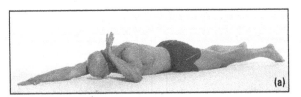

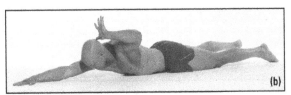

Photo by Jorge Alvarez, www.alvarezphoto.com

Twists and reaches

Figure 12-95 shows the starting and ending positions for twists and reaches.

Y-cuffs

Figure 12-96 shows the starting and ending positions for Y-cuffs.

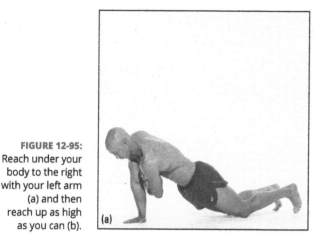
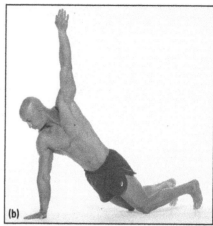

FIGURE 12-95: Reach under your body to the right with your left arm (a) and then reach up as high as you can (b).

Photo by Jorge Alvarez, www.alvarezphoto.com

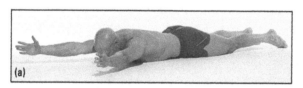
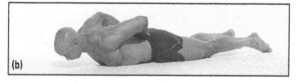

FIGURE 12-96: Reach your arms to the Y position with your thumbs up (a) and then place your hands on your lower back and raise your elbows (b).

Photo by Jorge Alvarez, www.alvarezphoto.com

TIP

Once you've completed this 13-week routine, or you want to be guided via video, head on over to marklauren.com, where we have, years of programs that hold your hand rep for rep and day by day. With routines like the Prep Program, Daily Workouts, and the 90-Day Challenge, you can progress smartly to much higher levels of fitness. Use promo code STRONG15 to save 15 percent on annual memberships. We also have a supportive and active community that you can join for free at community.marklauren.com.

4

Calisthenics for Special Circumstances

Chapter **13**

Doing Calisthenics When You're Pregnant

C alisthenics don't prepare you for a specific sport alone. They prepare you for life. And what more important thing to prepare for, than a new life itself? This chapter covers how to approach fitness before, during, and after pregnancy.

WARNING

It's always a good idea to check with your doctor before you begin an exercise regimen and that's even more true when you're exercising for two! Be sure you have the green light with your OB to exercise before exercising, especially if you are beginning a new regimen.

The Benefits of Exercise Before and After Baby

Every benefit that calisthenics play in the overall well-being of an individual are amplified with pregnancy. Bodyweight exercises can help a woman prepare for the physical and emotional changes that she experiences during pregnancy. The benefits of regular, but careful, exercise during this transformative period include improved strength, enhanced mood, and easier labor.

Exercise also improves your mental well-being. Again, is there any time that this could be more crucial, for you and your baby?

Regular physical activity helps curb excessive weight gain, reducing the risk of gestational diabetes, and improving overall metabolic health. Maintaining a healthy weight is crucial for the well-being of both the mother and the developing child.

Taking Heed and Taking It Slow

WARNING

It is essential for pregnant women to consult with their healthcare providers before starting or continuing an exercise routine during pregnancy. Risks include:

>> **Injury:** Engaging in high-impact activities or exercises that carry a risk of falls can increase the likelihood of injury to both the mother and the developing baby. Activities such as contact sports, skiing, or vigorous cardio exercises may pose a higher risk.

Also, pregnancy increases production of *relaxin*, a hormone that increases the elasticity of connective tissues. If your range of motion increases practically overnight, before you haven't had a chance to build strength in those end-range positions, it can be easy to get injured.

>> **Overheating:** Elevating core body temperature during exercise can be harmful to the fetus. Overheating has been linked to an increased risk of birth defects in early pregnancy and an increased risk of dehydration, preterm labor, and neural tube defects in later stages. It is important to avoid exercising in hot and humid environments, to stay hydrated, and to listen to your body's cues to prevent overheating.

>> **Preterm labor:** Intense exercise and excessive physical exertion may trigger contractions and potentially lead to preterm labor in some cases. It is important to be mindful of your body's limits and avoid pushing beyond what feels comfortable.

>> **Reduced blood flow to the uterus:** Certain exercises that involve lying flat on the back for prolonged periods, especially after the first trimester, can compress the inferior *vena cava* (a large vein) and reduce blood flow to the uterus. This can potentially affect fetal oxygen supply. It is advisable to avoid prolonged periods of lying flat on your back.

Preparing for a Successful Pregnancy and Delivery

Perhaps one of the greatest advantages of calisthenics is that they produce increased stamina and endurance, which can be advantageous during labor and delivery.

Getting fit before getting pregnant

Your ability to tolerate activity during pregnancy depends mostly on your level of fitness before pregnancy. Getting in shape before pregnancy improves pregnancy fitness (or preparedness), which affects your ability to adapt to the physical changes that occur during gestation.

During pregnancy isn't the best time to start an exercise program. But if you do, you should start with an extremely gentle workout program, designed with the help of your healthcare provider.

Volume over intensity

As mentioned, always consult your healthcare provider before beginning an exercise routine, especially during pregnancy. They can provide guidance as to what you individually can safely tolerate. Some obvious no-no's during pregnancy are activities that carry a risk of falls or hard impact.

As a general rule, it's best to focus on light exercise. If you need to progress in the difficulty of your activity, increase the amount of light exercise you do instead of increasing the difficulty or intensity of what you're doing.

As an example of increasing volume, instead of intensity, try increasing the frequency of your workouts instead of increasing the difficulty. Or try increasing the number of sets in a workout, instead of increasing the difficulty of the exercises.

If anything, take a step back into easier movements and simply increase their frequency if you feel you need more challenge.

Increased stress tolerance

Exercise can combat so many potentially negative side effects of pregnancy. For example, women often experience hormonal changes that can lead to mood swings and increased stress. But exercise releases endorphins — known as those "feel-good" hormones — which help counter stress, anxiety, and depression. They promote better sleep patterns, boost self-esteem, and enhance body image. They can also help expectant mothers adapt to the physical and emotional changes associated with pregnancy.

Indeed, from Day 1 of pregnancy, to birth, to motherhood, calisthenics can be there for you. Stronger muscles contribute to better posture, reduced back pain, and improved balance. This combats the physical stress of carrying around an extra person in your womb, and later in your arms.

The bodyweight exercises in this book help to strengthen the muscles needed for childbirth, such as the core, pelvic floor, and leg muscles. Then, because calisthenics boosts energy levels, it reduces the exhaustion that often accompanies the early stages of motherhood.

Improved recovery

Exercise improves your ability to recover from physically, mentally, and emotionally stressful situations. Pregnancy, childbirth, and motherhood are perhaps the most extreme of all three.

Healthy women are more likely to produce healthy babies. And the benefits don't stop there. After giving birth, calisthenics aid in postpartum recovery, restoring strength and energy, and promoting mental well-being.

REMEMBER

Ideally, it's best to be fit before pregnancy so that you can continue with safe and gentle exercise during your pregnancy and maintain your fitness as much as possible until childbirth.

The bodyweight exercises in this book help restore muscle tone, especially in the abdominal area, which can be weakened during pregnancy and childbirth. Strengthening these muscles can alleviate back pain, improve posture, and prevent issues such as urinary incontinence. Exercise also provides much-needed energy and combats postpartum fatigue. And, as always, exercise stimulates the production of endorphins, reducing symptoms of postpartum depression and promoting overall mental well-being.

While caring for a newborn can be the most time-demanding thing a person will ever do, dedicating time for your own personal physical activity can only help make it easier. Both you and your child need and deserve the strongest you.

Chapter **14**

Working Out with Limited Mobility

s you've learned by now, athletic performance depends primarily on positioning yourself properly, and that comes from ideal joint alignment. But what if you're unable to get into ideal joint alignment? Millions of people suffer from short-term, acute injuries, or cope with longer-term, chronic mobility issues. If you're one of them, working out improperly carries great risk.

In contrast, exercising properly with calisthenics can bring great rewards. This chapter talks about why it's important to adopt calisthenics into your life, even when (especially when!) you have issues with mobility. The exercises in this chapter can help you increase your overall mobility and feel better. Chapter 10 also contains exercises that can help improve your mobility.

Getting the Essentials Right

Moving in ideal joint alignment means moving through life as efficiently as possible. But when you can't get into ideal joint alignment in the first place, exercise becomes inefficient. Your body will often try to compensate by using its better functioning joints and limbs to pick up the slack.

Go back to the analogy in Chapter 1 about your body being a tower, it only stands up because of the guy lines (cords that hold the tower down). When they are all perfectly positioned and balanced, towers can withstand hurricanes and earthquakes.

Now imagine one guy line goes slack. If you strengthen and tighten the other guy lines in response, what happens to the tower? Your tower bends and leans in those directions. And if it doesn't tumble on its own, the next storm will send it crashing to the earth.

The irony is that far from making you healthier, trying to compensate by using your functioning joints and limbs to pick up the slack often leads to further injury. Your body will naturally do this without you even noticing, until too often it's too late.

The key to improving the strength of your body's tower is to start safely and then effectively build your athletic foundation.

Finding your safest starting point

The key is to regress to the safest starting point. Ideal alignment means you can be in positions where you can absorb force safely. Stress tolerance and athletic performance depend on, among other things, your ability to position your body correctly. Floor exercises are ideal for this. The front lying, side lying, back lying, and crawling movements make it easy to maintain good posture while training all the joint functions.

REMEMBER

Virtually everyone can do the floor exercises in this book. These are the workouts on Tuesday, Thursday, and Saturday in the 13-week exercise program. So start there. Keep all parts of your body straight and in perfect alignment as described and shown in the photos.

The only variable is your range of motion.

For example, if you only have a two-inch range of motion for Dirty Dogs, which develop external hip rotation, that's just fine. That's what you do.

The next week, maybe you get 2.5 inches, then 3 inches the following week, until eventually you get satisfactory, pain free range of motion. Range of motion differs for everyone. Your ultimate range of motion is whatever is satisfactory for you to move through life with optimal performance, pain free. That's your progression.

Keep practicing the floor exercises as long as you're improving and making gains. Usually this means going through the 13-week cycle two or three times. Then you can move onto the strength training workouts on Monday, Wednesday, Friday.

REMEMBER

The 13-week program in Chapter 12 was designed this way on purpose. Someone who's more advanced can do all six days of training per week, whereas someone with limited mobility should try three days on Tuesdays, Thursdays, and Saturdays. You'll get great results by sticking to the floor exercises for a couple of 13-week cycles until you're ready to start the more difficult workouts. Systematically training all the joint functions is an incredibly simple and effective way to eradicate pain and increase mobility.

THE ULTIMATE EXAMPLE OF CONQUERING LIMITED MOBILITY

A few years back, the rehabilitation center director at the Sport University of Cologne asked me to tour their center for children with cerebral palsy. I soon learned that it was considered the leading clinic in the world for children with permanent movement disorders. Many had no locomotion at all. The children spend all day training with renowned therapists, day in and day out. The care and technology these kids received amazed me. We paused our tour of the facility to watch a young boy named Fabien suspended in a monstrous, complex, computerized, sci-fi looking machine that made him walk, something he would never do on his own.

"But can he even get up off the ground?" I asked.

The director shook her head.

It was like having a machine force your hand to write calculus equations when you are still struggling with basic arithmetic.

The next day, they let me spend an hour with nine-year-old Fabien. I carried Fabien to a training mat and laid him on his side in a cradle position with his knees stacked and pulled up toward his chest. At first, he could barely lift his top knee off the bottom knee, which requires external hip rotation. But he was an extremely bright and motivated kid. We worked on this until he could open his legs quickly and actually resist me pushing down against his knee. After more isolated joint functions in lying positions, I got him rolling. We then worked movement by movement to get him from a front lying position to a crawling position. I showed him how to shift his weight to get his leg under him, and build up into a full crawling position. An hour later, I watched Fabien get up off ground by himself, for the first time in his life.

And I realized I just might be looking at the solution to the great fitness riddle. Because here it was: all the scientific complexities of functional strength training simplified to their most fundamental essence. By stripping away everything that wasn't needed, I'd put into practice what I believed were the common denominators of locomotion. And I watched a boy move in a way the world told him would never be possible.

How working with limited mobility inspired my program

Working with the kids at the rehabilitation center in Cologne was just too awesome. Their minds were sharp. Their wills were strong. They knew what they dreamed of doing with their bodies. But had never been shown how. So I flew back to Germany the next month, stayed longer at the clinic, and designed a program for them. I saw it time and again, these kids who had been unmotivated to do traditional strength training, eagerly practiced the movements I showed them. Because they intuitively knew they needed them. The reward is instant, which drives the needed behavior. Their reactions to newly conquered positions were like infants who sit up for the first time and sees the world from a new viewpoint.

It was the ultimate irony: Children with cerebral palsy were validating my methods for attaining peak athletic performance as quickly and easily as possible.

I wanted to put my methods to the test on the other extreme of the spectrum. So I went to work with the elderly in assisted living facilities. While the children in Cologne had never learned the fundamental athletic skills, the elderly had lost them. Their physical abilities were rapidly declining. When I got to one facility in Portland, they were playing with little pink dumbbells and doing water aerobics. Their trainers were simply trying to slow down the regression of their athletic skills. Father time is unstoppable, right?

By creating a progression out of the exact movements, I believe you need to transition between lying and standing positions. I trained an 84-year-old woman to get off the ground and walk without a cane for the first time in 20 years.

I realized that if I could teach these people to move in ways previously thought impossible, applying the same methodology, I could turn the everyday person into an athlete. And I soon began doing so. Because the everyday person's learning curve is far less steep, and their potential far greater.

This is how I learned to build the best bodies: by drilling only the movements that accurately duplicate what we need to move like athletes as efficiently as possible, and then stringing them together in progressions.

Getting and Staying Prepared for Life

Fitness requires preparation. The secret to reaching and maintaining your peak fitness lies in continually refining and improving the basics on which everything else is built. To reach your own peak performance, you should keep working on improving the floor exercises and transitions between lying, kneeling, and standing positions for the rest of your life.

There will never be a point at which you no longer need to train, because there's never a point at which you can afford to let your foundation deteriorate. The advanced athletes I've worked with still train these fundamental movements regularly, as should anyone with limited mobility. The only difference is that if you have limited mobility, you need to focus on the floor exercises and developmental movements first. Once you're sure on your feet and have a solid foundation, you can move to more difficult movements.

Getting up and down from the floor

Aside from improving joint function, these transitions are specifically what you need in order to move safely and confidently through life. It is in these transitions that we first learned to control weight shifting while developing the coordination, strength, and flexibility needed for more complex activities such as walking and playing sports. By regularly revisiting these movements, you can maintain the essentials needed to maintain your independence and well-being.

The risk of serious injury due to falling goes up as we age, often because we lose the athletic ability needed to control the transitions needed to move with ease between lying and standing positions. Keeping that foundation strong, can keep you not only living longer, but healthier and happier.

To improve these essential movement skills, practice the following transitions three times per week along with the floor exercises in the 13-week program.

Rolling exercises

With this simple exercise, you learn to move your arms around a neutral spine while shifting your weight laterally, which is also needed for much more complex movements, like sprinting and boxing. For more information about this exercise, see Chapter 5.

1. **Start in a back lying position, as shown in Figure 14-1a.**

2. **Roll to your left by reaching across your body with your right arm, as shown in Figure 14-1b.**

   You'll need to lift your head and perform a crunch in order to lift your chest, so you can roll.

3. **Get to a front lying position with your right arm under your right shoulders, as shown in Figure 14-1c, and then reverse the movement to complete the repetition.**

Perform four rolls to the left and four rolls to the right.

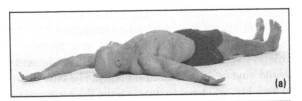
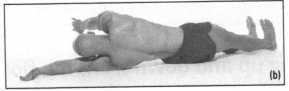
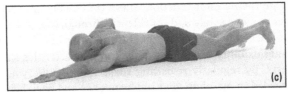

FIGURE 14-1: This simple rolling exercise helps tone your core.

Photo by Jorge Alvarez, www.alvarezphoto.com

REMEMBER

Use your abdominals to perform a crunch as you reach across your body to roll from a back lying position to a front lying position. Not only is this an extremely useful movement in real life, it's also a great core exercise.

Lying to kneeling transitions

This is a full-body movement that teaches you to transition smoothly from a front-lying position to a tall double-kneeling position. You'll develop useful strength while also improving your posture. For more information about this exercise, see Chapter 5.

1. **Start from a front lying position with your hands under your shoulders and knees on the ground, as shown in Figure 14-2a.**

2. **Walk your hands back until your hips are behind your knees, as shown in Figure 14-2b.**

3. **Get to a tall double-kneeling position, as shown in Figure 14-2c, and then reverse the movement to get back to a front lying position.**

Perform four transitions from front lying to double-kneeling.

TIP

Try adding a towel or pad under your knees if they are uncomfortable in the double-keeling position.

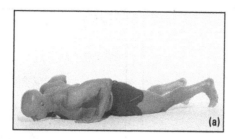
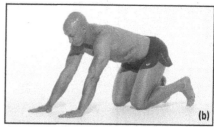
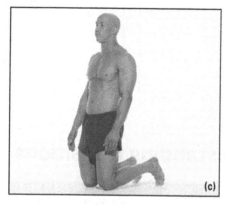

FIGURE 14-2:
Start in a front
lying position
with your hands
under shoulders
(a), push your
hips back past
your knees (b),
and get into a
double-kneeling
position (c).

Photo by Jorge Alvarez, www.alvarezphoto.com

Kneeling to standing transitions

This exercise is exceptional for developing strength, flexibility, and balance that's useful in real life. As mentioned, almost everything you do in life involves stepping. As you progress with this exercise, challenge yourself to take big lunging steps while maintaining a tall upright posture.

1. **From a tall double-kneeling position, shift your weight onto your right hip, and then step forward with the left leg into a single kneeling position, as shown in Figure 14-3a.**

2. **Shift your weight onto your left leg and get to a tall standing position, as shown in Figure 14-3b. Reverse the movement to complete the repetition.**

Perform four kneeling to standing transitions stepping forward with the left leg, and then perform four repetitions stepping forward with the right leg.

TIP

You don't have to keep your arms at the T position as shown in Figure 14-3. Instead, you can use your hands to support yourself by placing them on the knee of your forward leg. This helps especially on the way up. If you still struggle to transition between kneeling and standing positions, try using a sturdy surface such as a couch to assist yourself.

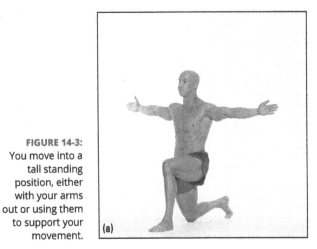 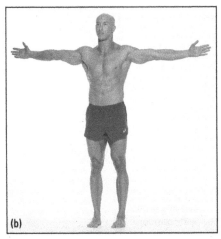

FIGURE 14-3:
You move into a
tall standing
position, either
with your arms
out or using them
to support your
movement.

(a) (b)

Photo by Jorge Alvarez, www.alvarezphoto.com

Back lying to standing transitions

Now it's time to put it all together! Note that this exercise is a progression of the following ones, so it's naturally more challenging. Take your time and don't get discouraged if you can't do this right off the bat.

1. **Start in a back lying position and roll onto your stomach.**

2. **Push your hips back and get to a double-kneeling position.**

3. **Step forward with the left leg and then stand up tall. Reverse the movement to complete the rep.**

Perform four repetitions by first rolling left and stepping forward with the left leg, and then do four repetitions on the right side.

If you're feeling strong and confident, you can add an extra step by transitioning to a standing position on a single leg, known as the *stork stance*, as shown in Figure 14-4.

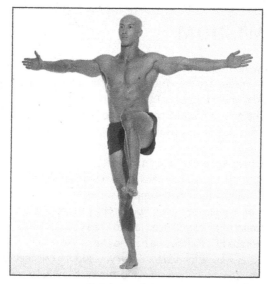

Photo by Jorge Alvarez, www.alvarezphoto.com

We're the Only Mammals That Walk on Two Feet

There only exist two mammals that can even *move* mostly on two feet. The other is the kangaroo. And honestly, they barely count because they often use their tails, like the third leg in a tripod, to balance.

Our species alone is a walking, talking towers of bones. We balance on the sticks of our legs, our feet being the only two points of contact with the ground. If a dogs have a weak leg, they limp.

If any part of us is out of balance or atrophied, it's amazing how difficult it becomes to stay upright. Anyone who's pulled a hamstring learns pretty quickly that we need every last joint function just to stand up. With a pulled hamstring, simply stepping a few inches to the side to steady yourself — something we do dozens of times a day without thinking — can send you to the ground with ten out of ten pain.

EASTERN WISDOM

In Southeast Asia, I've noticed that older people are more sure on their feet. There, 80 year-olds sit on the ground to rest. They'll sit in a squat for 45 minutes while they eat. They sit beautifully and effortlessly. Their posture is perfect. Their lines straight. Perfectly efficient. The men and women I've come to know there often don't experience the hip and back problems so many people in the Western world fall prey to.

But for many westerners, just sitting upright in a natural position can be humbling. As anyone who's sat through a ten-day meditation retreat knows, simply sitting cross-legged on a cushion, without back support, without moving, for an hour or more often causes excruciating pain. No matter how strong you are, myself included, it's incredible the functional muscles you need just to keep your spine upright without a chair. When for hundreds of millennia, we had no chairs. We rested and moved with our bodies the way they were intended to. When you adopt a calisthenics routine, you can return to that. You can return to resting and moving beautifully and effortlessly at any age.

It's incredible, how when one single connection is weakened, the entire kinetic chain is often compromised and you can develop unsafe and ineffective movement patterns that progressively lead to more serious injuries. For that reason, you have to avoid falling into the trap of avoidance strategies, where you start to do basic things in less than optimal ways in order to avoid the pain and discomfort. It's a vicious cycle that especially affects older populations, especially in Western cultures where developmental movements have been eroded from a lifetime of sitting in chairs.

Start small and progress gradually.

TIP

One of the most important qualities that improves with exercise is stress tolerance, which can also be described as work capacity. Especially when you're older, it often doesn't take much to make you sore and tired. Ideally, you want to avoid being very sore after exercising. Otherwise, you won't be able to exercise again in a day or two. And then there goes your consistency. And consistency is what leads to progress.

Chapter **15**

Starting Your Kids on Calisthenics

Kids learn from playing. But nowadays, for the first time in human history, a lot of the playing they do isn't in the physical world. It's on screens. That's why now more than ever, it's vital to take an active role in your children's fitness. It's not only fruitful, it's efficient: You spend quality time with your kids and strengthen your relationship and your bodies, all at the same time. And now, with this book, you only need a small space to do it.

This chapter discusses how to introduce your kids to fitness and train with them and explains why exercise is so important for growing bodies.

Keeping Your Kids Happy and Healthy with Movement

Incorporating calisthenics into a child's everyday life strengthens them both physically and mentally. Keeping it *enjoyable* promotes a positive attitude toward physical activity, and can lead to a lifelong fitness foundation.

And it keeps them happy, because physical activity releases hormones that lead to improved mood. Engaging in exercise also provides an outlet to release pent-up energy, reduces stress, and combat anxiety or boredom.

Furthermore, exercising with your kids is a great form of real-world social interaction. When family or friends workout together, they deepen their relationships and build teamworking skills. All of this contributes to a child's sense of belonging.

Leading by example and training together

There is no leadership technique more powerful than displaying the behavior you want to see in others. If you want your kids to be healthy and exercise regularly, the best way to influence them is to develop your own healthy exercise habits. That should start with calisthenics.

Unlike other forms of working out, calisthenics is already kid-friendly. Because these movements are virtually the safest and most functional for our bodies, there's virtually no exercise in this book that is unsafe for kids. But I hope it goes without saying by now, this is only as long as they carefully follow the steps for proper posture.

But first things first. Kids should start with the floor exercises in Chapter 4 to ensure they systematically develop all the joint functions for their hips, spine, and shoulders. Once they can properly execute those exercises, they'll be well prepared to start experimenting with the exercises in the remaining chapters of Part 2. If you want more guidance, simply follow the 13-week program in Chapter 12. Kids learn and adapt quickly, so don't be surprised if they are soon outperforming you.

PAVING THE WAY FOR A BRIGHTER, STRONGER FUTURE FOR ALL THOSE AROUND YOU

From talking to women all over the world about their fitness goals and their workout practices, it seems that one of the greatest obstacles to many of them developing a lean, strong body is a woman's reluctance to focus on her own needs. Between families and/or careers, many women are busier now than ever before. They are so focused on others that they have little time for themselves.

Here's what I find ironic: Giving so much of yourself to those around you may in fact be making life more difficult for them, not easier. Certainly that's the case when it comes to your long-term health. There's obviously unavoidable ailments that can come with aging. But some you can prevent, and staying physically fit puts you in the best situation for that. Don' you want to put yourself in the best position for your loved ones to visit you in your home rather than the hospital? Don't you want to do all you can to stay out of a wheelchair? Your focus on others at the expense of your own health perpetuates an endlessly repeating, zero sum game; no one wins. You spend time and energy taking care of others who later must spend their time and energy taking care of you. You have limited your life's potential so that they may have a good life, but then they too have to limit their potential, not only caring for the own offspring, but also caring for you.

While there is no actual fountain of youth, exercise is proven over and over again to be the closest thing. Becoming a stronger, leaner you *now* paves the way for a brighter, stronger future for all those around you. If you care about their happiness, care about your own. Then you can lead by example. And pave the way for a brighter future for the next generations too.

Instilling/encouraging the joy of movement

Make these exercise sessions fun for your kids. Don't force movement that they aren't ready for or can't do properly. It's much better at this point to instill a love of moving and playing than it is to force your children to bike a certain distance, do a sport they don't like, or run through an exhausting exercise regimen.

Of course, the best thing you can do is show your children how much you enjoy movement yourself, by exercising and playing joyfully with them.

Increasing your child's injury resistance

Giving your child the basic building blocks needed to move properly allows for optimal learning of physical fitness with reduced risk of injury.

Through exercise, children develop better coordination, balance, flexibility, and agility, which are crucial factors in preventing accidents like sprains and strains, and minimizing the severity of potential injuries.

Perhaps most important, calisthenics, if done properly, steers your child's body into proper alignment and posture. As early as elementary school, any keen observer can see the posture in too many children already weakening. Necks bend forward and shoulders hunch. These faults only worsen by the time they become teenagers and spend an inordinate amount of time bent over their smartphones and other devices.

By encouraging children to lead an active lifestyle, we empower them with the tools they need to build a resilient body, capable of withstanding the challenges and demands of their daily activities.

Learning to learn better

Athletic ability is learned like any other subject. When the fundamental building blocks are in place, it's much easier to learn everything else that is built on them. You can think of joint functions as the ABCs of movement. You need the entire alphabet if you're going to start writing. It's no different with your body.

For the purpose of developing basic athletic ability, the exercises in Chapter 4 are ideal. They systematically cover hip, spine, and shoulder functions in positions where it's easy to maintain good posture, so users can learn to move their arms and legs around a neutral spine.

Start with a light and playful approach with the intention of improving useful athletic skills, which are the floor exercises. You'll see rapid improvements with this approach, because better performance is largely the result of improved coordination. The minimum should be one set of four repetitions with each exercise. From there, progress gradually up to eight reps exercise. Once that's easy, you can go through all the exercises twice.

Proper posture and movement is indeed like learning a language. Learn it when you're very young, and you'll be fluent the rest of your life. Try to learn it later, and it takes years.

Simply having your kid go outside "to play" is a good first step, especially as a way to encourage a love of movement and the outdoors. But random playing does not usually develop all your joints and muscles in balance. Sure, you build strengths, but you also develop weaknesses in your fitness foundation. Ditto with sports, especially when kids become specialized in one or two of them. Supplementing even the most active child's lifestyle with calisthenics, such as the floor exercises or maybe even the entire 13-week program in this book, can help them succeed in organized sports and prevent injuries. Aligning your body and mastering the basics of human movement makes it much easier to learn more complex athletic skills and activities later.

TIP

And, here's the weird thing: You actually might be able to learn a thing or two from how your kids themselves move. Children possess an innate ability to problem solve. Often, they'll do movements more simply and efficiently than adults, like even just getting up off the ground. Kids can move in a natural way that many of the exercises in this book replicate. A way that many adults need to train hard to get back to.

Overcoming Complaints about Exercising

Behavior that gets rewarded is repeated. So it's vital, particularly with youngsters, to keep things positive and rewarding. Especially at the start, keep the workouts light and make sure there is some kind of payoff at the end of the session, even if it's simply a couple of high fives or a favorite snack.

Ideally, you want to develop an environment where your children fall in love with exercise and develop lasting fitness habits. That's way more useful to the child than trying to "toughen 'em up." The desire for harder workouts should evolve naturally out of the child's attachment to training, especially when they see the benefits that arise from it. That's why workouts should be appropriate for their fitness levels and not excessively hard.

TIP

Apply the acronym KIP: Keep it playful. Keep it positive. Keep it progressing.

MARK'S INSPIRING JOURNEY

Like many, body image first drove me to give this fitness thing a try. I was 13, a scrawny, shy kid, and I wanted to do something about it. I had no access to weights, so I did push-ups and sit-ups in my bedroom before dinner. Eventually, I could do 75 non-stop push-ups and 600 sit-ups. Then I did more. It can be hard to shape the world around you. But I found a way to shape the world within me. I soon became a stronger version of myself in every way. Confidence in all I did soared, including winning regional high school bodybuilding titles.

Many years later, at the Air Force's 22nd Special Tactics Squadron, I continued to use bodyweight exercises to keep myself physically fit and able to meet the extreme demands of airfield seizures, combat search and rescue, and reconnaissance and surveillance missions. It was there that I managed to break (and still hold) the U.S. military's record for the longest swim underwater (133 meters in two and a half minutes).

Then, five days before September 11, 2001, I left my team to become a full-time Military Physical Training Specialist. I was tasked with physically preparing the most elite Special Operations troops for immediate deployment into areas of forward combat operation.

Every six weeks, I got a new shipment of untrained recruits. Most came to me soft and weak. By the end of the course, they were lean, strong, and confident. By revamping the

(continued)

(continued)

physical training programs, I was able to produce better results with only a fraction of the time and fewer injuries. From SEALs to Green Berets, I proudly watched my trainees garner medals. I developed a purely bodyweight program that evolved until my squadrons were using it not only in the field, but even when equipment was available.

My journey from military trainer to international bestselling author was a dream come true. I've had the opportunity to train thousands of people, certify hundreds of trainers, and train the trainers of trainers. I've had a ringside seat beside the men and women at the forefront of elite training and sports science. But more than all the science I studied and the research I conducted, experience inspired me most: from Dubai to Laos, from Afghanistan to Portland. I worked hard to build a training method superior to any other in developing muscular, lean, physically fit bodies as fast as possible. And now I share it with you.

When a child gets into shape for the first time, it changes their whole life. The confidence born from performing well, competing, and yes, looking good among your peers, can extend into all areas of a child's development.

When you become a parent, let that be your primary motivator to exercise. It's a reason to look, feel, and perform your best. Be a role model. You owe it to those around you as much as you owe it to yourself. And often the easiest way to exercise yourself is to exercise with your children.

Chapter **16**

Nine-Minute Workouts

K eep what gets results best and chuck the rest. Reducing training to only the most essential bodyweight movements nearly eliminates the need to spend time and money while increasing your returns. Just like many professional athletes do, you'll attain the most strength and the leanest body through the movements most vital to our survival.

The nine-minute workouts in this chapter help you conquer three of the main reasons people give for not exercising:

» I do not have time.

» I cannot afford equipment or gym memberships.

» I do not have enough space.

We can all find nine minutes. I know a truck driver who pulls over and throws down a camping mat at a rest stop once a day. A few minutes later he's driving off, fitter than he was just ten minutes earlier. And, since they increase energy and focus, the minutes you sacrifice to execute these exercises several times a week will make many other things in your life quicker and more efficient.

For more guidance on how to use these exercises in a routine, check out the 13-week program in Chapter 12. You can also find many more exercise programs for varying fitness levels, as well as video tutorials, via the marklauren.com website. Use promo code STRONG15 to save 15 percent on annual memberships.

Athleticism Leads to Efficiency

These nine-minute workouts drill only the movements that accurately duplicate what you need to move as efficiently as possible and then string them together. They combine the isolated functions of your joints into whole body movements, and then merge these whole body exercises into dynamic, flowing movements that and strengthen your entire body.

For those seeking to lose fat, it's incredibly inefficient to exercise for the sake of burning calories. An hour on a treadmill can be undone by a slice of bread. So it's a lot more efficient just to eat a little less. And build power and speed with this program. The increased muscle will burn fuel (calories), even while you sleep. And if you're worried about cardiovascular conditioning, this nine-minute program will build that too.

No matter what your current fitness level, everyone will see gains from following this program. If you're just starting out, the amount of reps you can accomplish in the time allotted will increase over time. You can build a better physique by practicing the skills to perform these exercises properly. Then you'll be astonished how quickly you'll progress into advanced levels.

Structuring Your Workouts

Each exercise in this plan prepares you for the next. Each nine-minute workout day also prepares you for the next. Plan on progressing from three to five times a week in six-week cycles.

The movements are split into the three basic categories:

>> Pushing exercises

>> Pulling exercises

>> Hip hinging exercises

Each workout includes exercises from each of these categories, ensuring that every nine-minute routine trains your entire body top to bottom.

As mentioned, the program is broken up into six-week cycles. Just as each day builds on the last, each cycle builds more strength and skills than the last. You begin with Cycle 1 and progress all the way up to Cycle 4. After that, you can repeat Cycles 3 and 4 endlessly. You'll still be making gains because you'll find that you are be able to do more reps of each exercise.

Table 16-1 shows a matrix of the nine strength training exercises that are split into three categories for pushing, pulling, and hip hinging. Each of these categories includes three exercises. To make a nine-minute workout, choose one movement from each of the three categories. You can combine exercises from the different categories however you want, just make sure you have one from each category.

TIP

These workouts are best with a timer. Just make sure your phone screen doesn't go to sleep on you.

TABLE 16-1:

The Nine-Minute Exercise Matrix

Pushing	Pulling	Hip Hinging
Push-ups	Let-me-ins	Squats w/arms at T
Military press	Let-me-ups (knees bent)	Romanian deadlifts
DF glide	Let-me-ups (legs elevated)	Back lunges

After a quick warm up, you do one minute of your chosen pushing exercise, followed by one minute of your pulling exercise, followed by one minute of your hip hinging exercise. You then repeat that circuit two more times. That makes nine minutes total.

Workouts start with 40/20 intervals, meaning that you'll do each exercise for 40 seconds and then rest for 20 seconds. Then progress to 45/15, 50/10, and eventually to full one-minute work intervals without resting. A small decrease in your rest time can leads to a huge increase in your percentage of work time.

The interval approach is the most efficient method and provides enough progression, consistency, and variety to build full body workouts that apply enough stress to make you stronger.

Go easy when starting these workouts. No one is watching, so there's no one to impress. Use the easiest 40/20 work to rest intervals and pick exercise variations that you can do with good form even when you're fatigued.

Learn to pace yourself. Rather than going hard on a set to complete failure and then being useless for the remainder of the work interval, find a sustainable pace and take short breaks every few reps. This will increase the quality and quantity of your work. An example of pacing yourself is doing four reps and then taking a two-breath break before repeating. Adjust your pace as needed to keep yourself working throughout the duration of each work interval.

Starting with the Pushing Exercises

This section explains the three pushing exercises that you can use to build nine-minute workouts (push-ups, military presses, and DF glides). Keep in mind that each of these exercises has variations to make the movements easier or harder.

With that said, a simple way to perform difficult pushing exercises is to focus on controlling the downward portion of the movement and then "cheat" yourself back up into the starting position. You can learn a lot more about these exercises in Chapter 8.

Push-ups

The key to doing push-ups properly is getting a full range of motion while maintaining a straight body position from head to heels. If you need to, you can start with your knees on the ground (also called modified push-ups or knee push-ups) — still a good workout!

To make yourself straight, in any position, lightly flex your glutes and abdominals while lifting your chest slightly. Lastly, position your head so that your neck is relatively straight, as shown in Figure 16-1.

FIGURE 16-1:
Push-ups work the triceps, pectoral (chest) muscles, and shoulders.

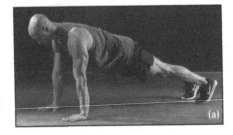
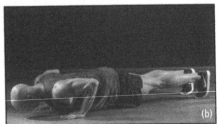

Photo by Jorge Alvarez, www.alvarezphoto.com

Military presses

The military press, shown in Figure 16-2, works the triceps and the delts. Your elbows shouldn't flair out completely and they shouldn't be completely tucked. They should be somewhere in the middle.

You can make this exercise a little easier by placing your hands on an elevated surface.

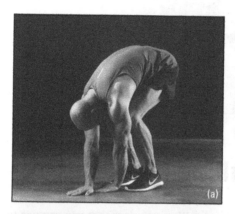
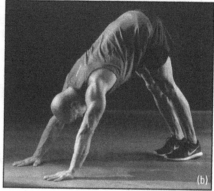
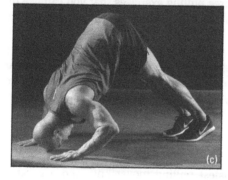

FIGURE 16-2: Place your hands on the ground shoulder width apart and lower your head between your hands.

Photo by Jorge Alvarez, www.alvarezphoto.com

DF glides

Think of this exercise as a push-up where you push your hips up into the air to get a good stretch after every rep. (DF stands for *dorsiflexion*, the backward bending of your foot or hand.)

To make this exercise easier, worm yourself up to the starting position of a push-up, and then bring your hips up into the air. Focus on a controlled descent with a long, straight body position at the end. Figure 16-3 shows the progression.

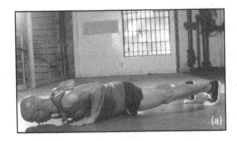
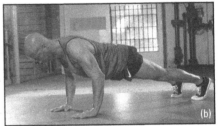
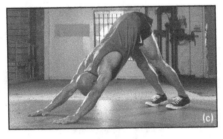

FIGURE 16-3:
This exercise adds to the classic push-up to evenly develop your chest, shoulders, and triceps.

Trying Out the Pulling Exercises

This section explains three pulling exercises that you can use to build your nine-minute workout. You can find more about these exercises in Chapter 9.

WARNING

There's plenty of room for creativity when finding places to do pulling exercises, such as going to a playground to use the monkey bars or using a tree, desk, door, or suspension straps, but use some common sense and good judgment. Be sure that the object is sturdy enough to easily support your weight!

Let-me-ins

Let-me-ins are the easiest pulling movements and a great starting place for beginners. Remember that you can wrap a hand towel around a door handle, railing, or anything else sturdy enough to support your weight. Figure 16-4 demonstrates this exercise.

Let-me-ups (knees bent)

Once you're able to do let-me-ins fairly easily, you're ready to start working with let-me-ups. These are pulling movements where your arms are perpendicular to your body. However, with let-me-ups, your body is horizontal instead of vertical. Keeping your knees bent makes the exercise easier. See Figure 16-5.

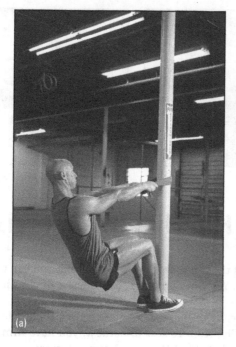
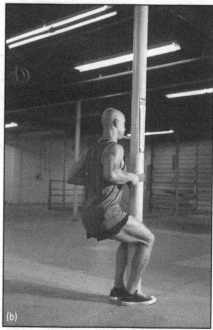

FIGURE 16-4:
Pull your chest to your hands and squeeze your shoulder blades together.

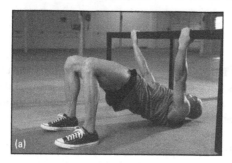
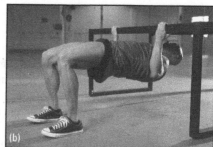

FIGURE 16-5:
Let-me-ups have plenty of variations that allow you to scale the difficulty for long-term progression.

Let-me-ups (legs straight)

Let-me-ups with your legs straight out in front of you are more challenging, because more of your weight is supported by your arms, rather than your legs (see Figure 16-6). Once you've master the bent-knee let-me-up, you're ready to move on to these!

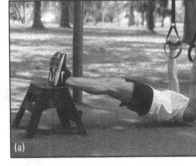
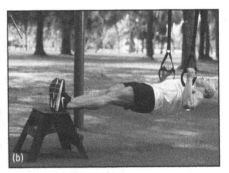

FIGURE 16-6:
Make yourself
straight head to
heels (a) and then
pull yourself up
between your
hands (b).

(a)

(b)

Photo by Jorge Alvarez, www.alvarezphoto.com

Moving on to the Hip Hinging Exercises

This section describes three hip hinging exercises that you can use to build your nine-minute workout. You can find more about these exercises in Chapter 7.

REMEMBER

You can vary the difficulty of these standing exercises slightly be using different arm positions. Typically, from easiest to hardest, you have Arms Front (zombie style), Arms at T, Hands Behind Head, and Arms straight over your head. Each position requires progressively more mobility and balance.

Squats

Figure 16-7 shows the T position squat. Performing squats with your arms at the T position strengthens your upper back, opens your chest, and challenges your ankle mobility. They key is to maintain perfect alignment even if it means using a relatively short range of motion.

REMEMBER

Stand with your feet hip-width apart and push your hips back bend your knees as if you're sitting onto a chair. As you sit back, lift your chest up and keep your toes and knees pointing straight ahead. Challenge yourself to go as deep as you can while maintaining correct alignment. Then stand up tall and straight before repeating.

For an easier variation, try holding your arms in the front zombie style, as shown in Figure 16-8.

TIP

There are many variations of the squat, including narrow squats, wide squats, overhead squats, one-legged squats, and more. See Chapter 7 for much more about squatting.

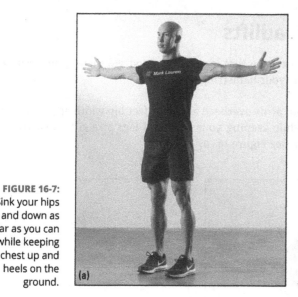

FIGURE 16-7: Sink your hips back and down as far as you can while keeping your chest up and heels on the ground.

(a) (b)

Photo by Jorge Alvarez, www.alvarezphoto.com

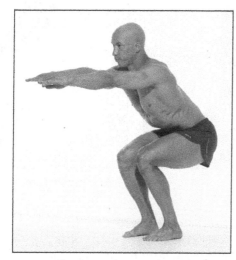

FIGURE 16-8: Squatting with your arms out in front of you is slightly easier than the T squat.

Photo by Jorge Alvarez, www.alvarezphoto.com

Romanian deadlifts

This is an exceptional exercise that lengthens and strengthens your entire body head to heels, especially your hamstrings.

To do it, stand with your arms overhead and your feet hip width apart. Point your toes straight ahead. While keeping your back and legs straight, push your hips back and bend forward. See Figure 16-9.

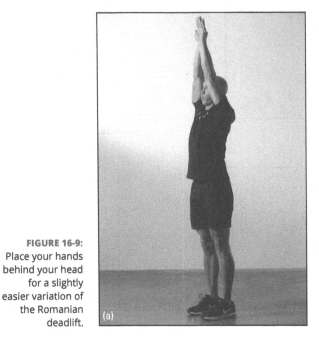
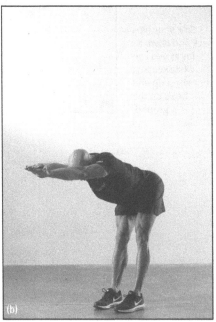

Photo by Jorge Alvarez, www.alvarezphoto.com

FIGURE 16-9: Place your hands behind your head for a slightly easier variation of the Romanian deadlift.

Back lunges

The back lunge is the best way to learn lunging movements, because stepping to the rear automatically pulls your hip back away from your feet, which puts you into better alignment to safely absorb the force.

Squats are more balanced than lunges, and lunges need more coordination. Some experts in the fitness world think it's better for beginners to start with squats. Also, lunges are not a good idea for anyone with knee pain. If this describes you, try squats instead.

To begin, stand with your feet hip-width apart and toes pointing straight ahead. Then take a big step back and lower your trailing knee, as shown in Figure 16-10.

FIGURE 16-10: You can make lunges easier by placing your hands on your hips.

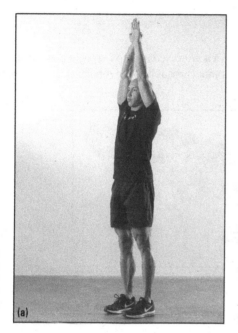

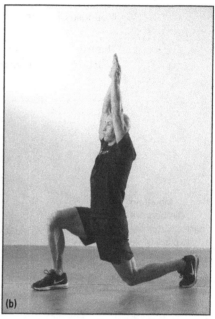

Photo by Jorge Alvarez, www.alvarezphoto.com

NINE-MINUTE WORKOUTS TO TONE AND TIGHTEN

This bonus section includes are three movements that you'll do for three rounds to make a nine-minute workout that'll blast the front and sides of your midsection. Perform each movement for 40 seconds followed by a 20-second rest period before moving on to the next exercise.

Mountain climbers

This exercise is as simple as it is effective. Get into a straight push-up position and alternate bringing your knees to your chest as if you're running in place while planking.

Mountain climbers are basically running in place while planking.

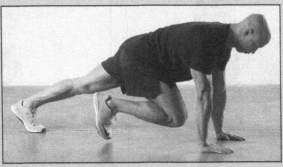

Photo by Jorge Alvarez, www.alvarezphoto.com

Side v-ups (right and left)

Side v-ups work the sides of your core. Finish one set lying on your left side. Then rest before doing another set lying on your right side.

1. **Lie on your left side with your left arm on the floor in front of you. Place your right hand on your head and lift your legs off the ground slightly.**

2. **While keeping your legs together, bring your knees to your right elbow.**

3. **Reset to the starting position to complete one rep.**

This exercise requires a bit of coordination, so be patient. It gets much easier once you get a feel for the timing of things.

Repeat these, but lying on your right side this time.

Side v-ups starting position (a) and ending position (b).

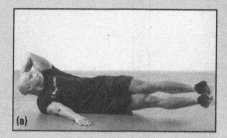 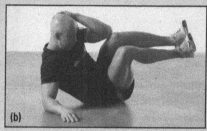

Photo by Jorge Alvarez, www.alvarezphoto.com

NINE-MINUTE GLUTE WORKOUT

In this bonus section, you're doing three movements for three rounds to make a nine-minute workout that primarily works your rear end or glutes. Practice each movement for 40 seconds followed by a 20-second rest period before moving on to the next exercise.

Wide squats

This is an excellent squatting variation for developing your gluteus maximus, which is the biggest part of your glutes.

1. **Stand tall and straight with your feet slightly wider than shoulder width apart. Your toes should be pointing straight ahead.**

2. **Push your hips back and bend your knees, as if sitting on a chair behind you.**

3. **Once your hips are knee height, squeeze your glutes to stand tall and straight.**

(continued)

(continued)

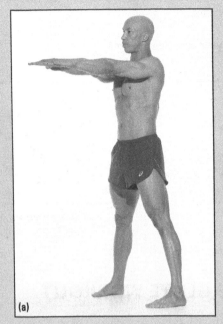 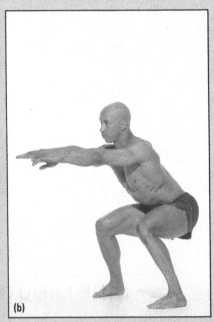

Wide squats starting position (a) and ending position (b).

Photo by Jorge Alvarez, www.alvarezphoto.com

Hip circles

Hip circles are great improving hip mobility while working the upper part of your glutes.

1. **Get into a crawling position and lift the left leg off the ground slightly.**

2. **Make big circles with the left knee going in a backward motion.**

Do the hip circles first with your left leg and then with your right.

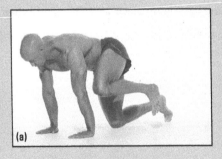 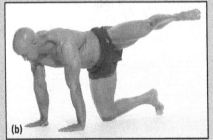

Make large backward circles with your left knee, getting your knee as high as is comfortable.

Photo by Jorge Alvarez, www.alvarezphoto.com

5

The Part of Tens

Chapter **17**

Ten Tips for Success

Stay Consistent

Generally speaking, you'll make much better gains with small frequent workouts than you will with big infrequent workouts. This is partly why bodyweight exercise is so incredibly effective. This book eliminates the unnecessary and focuses on the essentials, so you get more for less.

TIP

For specific guidance on how to use these exercises in a routine, check out the 13-week program in Chapter 12. You can also find many more exercise programs for varying fitness levels, as well as video tutorials, via the marklauren.com website. Use promo code STRONG15 to save 15 percent on annual memberships.

Schedule Your Workouts

The perfect time to work out will rarely fall into your lap. You need to make time. So look at your schedule and listen to your body.

If working out in the morning gets your blood flowing and energizes you for the rest of the day, make that time. Sleep is hugely important to your mental and physical well-being. So getting to bed on time is vital.

Some people hate working out in the morning! If that's the case, try fitting a few minutes of exercise into your lunch break, your afternoon, or your evening. And stick to that time every day. It'll soon become second nature. Chapter 16 has several nine-minute exercise routines you can choose from.

Listen to Your Body

Only *you* know what you need and when you need it. Only *you* feel your muscles, lungs, bones, and ligaments. In the end, only *you* can get you into shape. And that's all you need: You.

So much of what people have learned about fitness only hinders their potential. Unrealistic expectations, "no pain, no gain," pushing to injury, and more. Don't let fear of dumbbells, machines, or gadgets prevent you from reaching your optimum level of fitness. You don't need them!

Strengthen Your Weak Side First

If one arm is weaker than the other, give it the advantage of starting with it first, when possible. Doing exercises a single limb at a time is one of the most effective ways to build all the components of fitness. Not only does it correct any imbalance that goes unnoticed when both limbs are working at the same time, but one limb working alone has more than half the power of both limbs moving together. This is because when you work both limbs at the same time a defense mechanism (called the *bilateral deficit*) kicks in, hampering some of your motor units in an effort to prevent injury to your body during your heaviest lifts.

Rest and Recuperate

Remember, your body changes not while you work out, but while you rest. Getting seven-eight hours of sleep is also paramount. Train hard, but train smart. Leave yourself valuable time to recover. You'll come back physically and mentally refreshed if you do.

Don't Do Too Much

With a well-designed program, about 90 minutes or less of strength training a *week* is all that's needed for many novice and advanced athletes alike.

Any activities beyond this should be either light ones to aid recovery, or sport specific — for example, soccer practice if you play soccer. Working out more than is necessary only prolongs recovery and slows progress.

Show Up

As with many things, the hardest part is often getting started. Next time you don't feel like training, try tricking yourself: Tell yourself that you're just going to do a few sets. What you'll find is that usually, after you get warmed-up, you start feeling better, your energy surges, and those few sets turn into a full-blown workout. Worst case, you end up with an abbreviated workout. It's still better than doing nothing!

Keep a Playful Mindset

Heck, if you're really not feeling it, just play around with some exercises. It doesn't always have to be so structured or serious. The great thing is that you don't even have to leave the room you're in. Just drop down and do some dive bombers (see Chapter 8), or lie under your desk and crank out some let-me-ups (Chapter 9), or grab a railing and start some let-me-ins (Chapter 9). I often have workouts where all I do is play around with different exercises. Have fun with it.

Count Your Wins, Not Your Losses

Even Delta Force, arguably the most elite (and clandestine) military unit in the world, only counts the people they save, not those lost. Focusing on your successes helps you keep a positive attitude.

Taking care of your body is a decision you make each day. So congratulate yourself when you can do one more rep than last week. Or when you can properly execute a new movement you couldn't before. You're literally changing yourself for the better.

Eat a Healthy Post-Workout Meal

After your workout, you have a small window of time — about 45 minutes — when your muscles are especially receptive to nutrients needed for recovery. Because you've caused micro-damage to your muscle fibers and depleted their sugar stores, they hunger for protein and carbs.

TIP

Depending on your weight, shoot for 50-175 grams of protein daily. And pair that with 200–300 grams of carbs per day.

Post-workout meals are the one time that you do not want to add fat to your shake or meal, since fat will slow the absorption of carbs and therefore blunt the insulin reaction, slowing the rate at which the muscles are resupplied the needed nutrients to begin repair and growth.

Chapter **18**

Ten Bodyweight Training Myths

Men and Women Should Train Differently

Women's muscles are composed of the same fibers as men's. The only difference is usually quantity, due to hormones.

There is no reason to train differently based purely on your gender. All genders gain and lose muscle and fat the same way. It's true, men and women often have different goals. But surprisingly, these different goals can be achieved with the same program.

Most women aren't looking to develop big chests and arms, but rather to firm and tone their entire body, especially their legs and glutes, which tend to be the hardest things to maintain as they age. The ironic thing is that they should do exactly the same thing to achieve these goals as men should do to bulk up.

If women exercise their upper bodies as much as their lower, their tummies would just be that much flatter, and their glutes that much tighter, because they would be increasing their overall lean muscle mass. Building and maintaining muscle, alone, is the most effective way to burn fat and calories.

In contrast, the manly man has been taught to hit the bench press, lat pull down machine, squat rack, and other contraptions of bodybuilding. However, this approach leads to less functional results than the full array of bodyweight exercises.

Women's Muscles Will Get Too Big If You Do Strength Training

"I don't want to get too muscular." This is a common concern we hear from women all over the world. Some have seen the initial results of strength training and then shied away in fear of becoming the next Ms. Olympia.

Just FYI, male and female professional bodybuilders (and likely some of the bigger guys at your gym) use steroids and other illegal substances. The human body — yours included — simply will not accrue that kind of muscle mass without serious drugs.

For men and women, the initial gains in muscularity that are common within the first couple of weeks of strength training are largely due to an increase in circulation within the muscles. Similarly, the jumps in strength are mostly due to the body's neurological adaptation to new movements rather than added muscle mass.

The fear that you will accidentally become more muscular than you intended or that you will start growing uncontrollably is unfounded. For women, consistently gaining a half pound of muscle a month is outstanding progress. For men, a pound and a half is comparable. Keep in mind that this will occur under ideal conditions. A muscular body is built through consistent dedication to strength training and proper nutrition. It won't happen overnight or accidentally.

You Can Reshape a Muscle by Doing Isolation Exercises

Your muscles can only get bigger or smaller. The shape that your muscles take, as they change in size, is largely determined by genetics.

Keep in mind though, that some muscle groups that we often think of as single muscles, such as the shoulders, thighs, or back, can be changed by emphasizing a certain muscle within that muscle group.

The shoulders, for example, can get that nice heart shape, when viewed from the side, by working the rear deltoid. But the shape that your rear deltoid takes is controlled to a large degree by genetics.

You Need High Reps for Definition and Low Reps for Mass

Neither your body nor a particular muscle will become more defined by doing a high amount of repetitions of any exercise as opposed to doing low repetitions. Your muscles can only get bigger or smaller. Starting to notice a theme here?

It's true that low rep workouts, consisting of powerful and explosive movements, will build more size (but not less definition) than high rep workouts, because the "fast twitch" muscle fibers required in explosive movements are much larger than "slow twitch" fibers required for more enduring tasks. But really, for mass, wouldn't you want to recruit all possible muscle fibers and not just the fast twitch?

Likewise, for "definition" — that is, losing body fat so the striations in your muscles show more — wouldn't you want to recruit all possible muscle fibers? Especially since the number one factor we have control over that affects our resting metabolic rate, and thus fat loss, is . . . yup, you guessed it . . . muscle mass!

Muscle Can Turn Into Fat

Fat cells and muscle cells perform completely different and separate functions, and one will never transform into the other. When someone becomes "soft" and overweight after being "hard" and muscular, it is because their calorie output no longer exceeds the calorie intake. Largely, this is due to a decreased metabolic rate from the loss of muscle. The loss of muscle is caused by the lack of necessary stimulus. There is no magical transformation of muscle into fat, just a loss of muscle mass and an increase of body fat.

You Can't Build Muscle and Lose Fat at the Same Time

If you're just beginning this program after a long period without much exercise, with proper nutrition, you'll experience gains in strength while losing fat at the same time. For more advanced athletes, it's tough, but not impossible. With a perfect balance of complex carbs, good fats, and enough protein, your body can achieve these seemingly separate goals.

Going Hungry Means Looking Healthy

People often starve themselves in order to lose weight. That's a no-go.

The body is very resourceful, and it will slow down its metabolic rate in order to compensate for the lack of calories. It tries to hold onto every calorie you consume, since it is unsure when it will be fed again. Then, once you resume your normal caloric intake, your metabolic rate remains slowed down. This is why people who try restrictive diets usually gain their original weight back and often some more too.

REMEMBER

The good news is that if you want to lose weight, you should never be starving. A well-balanced diet consisting of small frequent meals (every 2.5 to 3.5 hours) can lead to long-term success.

Exercise Machines Were Built for You

You're not a cyborg. You don't need machines to move your muscles through a fixed range of motion. Besides improving strength, endurance, and body composition, your training should develop stability, effective movement patterns, and coordination. By using gadgets that force you through a set motion, none of these latter qualities are improved.

Many Nautilus-type machines can even open you to injuries, because they often begin movements in the most vulnerable position. Consider a pec deck or preacher curl. Both begin the movement with your isolated working muscles fully stretched. Then they force you through a fixed motion that you'll likely never use in the real world. This is especially hazardous under heavy loads. Because your body is not functioning naturally, as a cohesive whole, ineffective motor patterns are developed, making you more susceptible to injury.

Bodyweight Exercises Don't Allow You to Adjust the Difficulty

Here are four simple ways of changing the difficulty of an exercise without adding weight:

>> Increase or decrease the amount of leverage.

>> Perform an exercise on an unstable platform.

>> Use pauses at the beginning, end, and/or middle of a movement.

>> Turn an exercise into a single limb movement.

Again, let's take the push-up, a standard exercise that works your chest, shoulders, triceps, abs, obliques, and lower back (unlike benching, which works half of these). If you do push-ups standing up with your hands against a wall a couple of feet in front of you, the exercise is pretty easy. Then try them with your hands on an elevated surface, like the edge of a bureau or windowsill. The lower the surface you use — a desk, a couch, a coffee table — the harder they get. Putting your hands on the floor, like a standard push-up, is harder. If you put your feet on the coffee table and your hands on the ground, the exercise becomes significantly more difficult. This is using *leverage* to increase the exercise's difficulty.

To make the exercise still harder you can place your hands on one or two balls, like a basketball. Now you're using an *unstable surface.*

Still harder is to do basketball push-ups with pauses at the bottom. Still not hard enough? Try doing them one-handed on the floor. Then one-handed with your feet on the couch. Then on an unstable surface. Then with pauses . . . You get the idea.

You've just gone from one variation of an exercise, that probably *everyone* reading this book can do, to a more difficult variation that probably *no one* reading this book can do right off the bat. The difficulty of bodyweight exercises can be tailored to suit the needs of virtually anyone. You have total control of the resistance.

Aerobics or "Cardio" Is the Only Way to Burn Calories

Here's the skinny: One pound of fat can fuel a 130-pound female for 15 hours at target "cardio" heart range. If simply moving our bodies around shed pounds, we would have wasted away to nothing long ago. We certainly never would survived the Ice Age.

More bad news for aerobic activity: Whether it's running, cycling, or a step class, one reason it gets easier the more you do it, is not because of improved cardiovascular conditioning, but because of improved economy of motion. Your body becomes more efficient at that particular movement. Wasted movements are eliminated, necessary movements are refined, and muscles that don't need to be tensed are relaxed and eventually atrophied.

Whether you want to lose fat, gain muscle, or do both, strength training should be the core of your conditioning.

Index

A

A frames, 160–161
abdominal exercises
  bodyrocks, 72–73
  hanging leg lifts, 79, 80
  jack knives, 84
  mountain climbers, 76
  mountain climbers across, 76–77
  mountain climbers around, 77–78
  parallel leg crunches, 80–81
  pillar reaches, 74–75
  reaching bodyrocks, 73
  rollouts, 78–79
  scorpion kicks, 79, 80
  side reaching bodyrocks, 73–74
  sit-ups, 83
  starfish crunches, 82
  tripod scissor kicks, 75
  V-ups, 83–84
abilities built through calisthenics, 12–14
active recovery, in 13-week program
  Friday, 244–245
  Monday, 237–238
  overview, 236
  Saturday, 245–247
  Thursday, 242–243
  Tuesday, 238–240
  Wednesday, 240–242
active recovery, overview, 196
adapting workouts for long-term progress, 193–195
aerobics versus strength training, 296
aging, avoiding disability in, 25, 266–267
AMRAP workouts, in 13-week program
  Block 1 (weeks 1-4), 204–206
  Block 2 (weeks 5-8), 216–218
  Block 3 (weeks 9-12), 228–230
  overview, 198–199
Archer push-ups, 130–131
arm circles, 160
assisted pull-ups, 154–155
athletic skills, learning in childhood, 268
attention, focusing, 28

B

back, strength training for. *See* pulling exercises
back lunges
  general discussion, 107
  nine minute workouts, 280–281
  in 13-week program
    in Block 1 of, 204, 205
    in Block 2 of, 217–218
back lying exercises
  back lying to standing transitions, with limited mobility, 262–263
  dead bugs, 45–46
  glute hip-ups, 46–47
  in 13-week program
    active recovery week, 237–238, 242–243
    in Block 1 of, 203–204
    in Block 2 of, 214–216
    in Block 3 of, 226–228
  up and overs, 47–48
  windshield wipers, 48–49
backpacks, using for strength training, 14
balance, 14
bear crawls, 141–142
bench, getting off of, 12
bicep curls, equipment for, 14
biceps, strength training for. *See* pulling exercises
bilateral deficit, 288
bloomers, 163–165
bodyrocks, 72–73, 201
bodyweight exercises. *See* calisthenics
bodyweight training myths, 291–296
Bosu ball, 17
bottom squats, 117–118, 119
bouncing push-ups, 135–136
breathing, focusing on, 28
Bulgarian split squats, 104–105

C

calisthenics. *See also* children, calisthenics for
  abilities built through, 12–14
  advantages of, 8–10
  for all bodies and abilities, 7–8
  basic exercise terms, 27–28
  benefits of exercise, 18
  bodyweight training myths, 291–296
  focusing on attention and breathing, 28
  gear for, 14–18
  getting comfortable with, 12
  in pregnancy, 251–254
  results from, 10–11

caloric intake, 294

cardiovascular endurance, 13

cardiovascular exercise versus strength training, 296

cerbral palsy, functional training in children with, 257–258

chairs, 16

chest exercises. *See* pushing exercises

children, calisthenics for
complaints, overcoming, 269–270
future benefits, 266–267
injury resistance, increasing, 267–268
leading by example and training together, 266
learning athletic skills, 268
overview, 265
positive attitude towards movement, instilling, 267

circuit training
in 13-week program
in Block 1 of, 208–210
in Block 2 of, 220–222
in Block 3 of, 232–234
overview, 199–200
general discussion, 189

classic push-ups, 128–130

clothing for workout, 18

complaints from children, overcoming, 269–270

consistency of workouts, 194, 287

Contra presses, 131–132

cool downs, 195–196

coordinated hip and shoulder exercises
kneeling to standing exercises, 67
lying to kneeling exercises, 65–66
from lying to stork stance exercises, 68–69
rolling exercises, 64–65

coordination, improving, 13–14, 26, 44

core strengthening exercises
abdominal exercises
bodyrocks, 72–73
hanging leg lifts, 79, 80
jack knives, 84
mountain climbers, 76
mountain climbers across, 76–77
mountain climbers around, 77–78
parallel leg crunches, 80–81
pillar reaches, 74–75
reaching bodyrocks, 73
rollouts, 78–79
scorpion kicks, 79, 80
side reaching bodyrocks, 73–74
sit-ups, 83
starfish crunches, 82
tripod scissor kicks, 75
V-ups, 83–84
lateral stability exercises
ITB kickouts, 87
ITB leg lifts, 86
overview, 84
side plank, 85
side V-ups, 85–86
lower back exercises
overview, 87
reverse hypers, 88
skydivers, 89–90
swimmers, 88–89
overview, 71

Cossack squats, 118–120

counting wins not losses, 289–290

crawling exercises
dirty dogs, 49
hip circles, 50
pointers, 51
straight wide legs, 52

in 13-week program
in active recovery, 238–240, 244–245
in Block 1 of, 206–208
in Block 2 of, 218–220
in Block 3 of, 230–232

cross steps, 122–123

cycles, defined, 27

D

dead bugs
general discussion, 45–46
in 13-week program
in active recovery, 237, 242
in Block 1 of, 203
in Block 2 of, 214–215
in Block 3 of, 226

deadlifts, 92–93

deadlifts to squats, 100–102, 230

deep squats, 165, 217

definition, reps for, 293

developmental movements, 23–25
coordinated hip and shoulder exercises
kneeling to standing exercises, 67
lying to kneeling exercises, 65–66
from lying to stork stance exercises, 68–69
rolling exercises, 64–65
overview, 63–64
weight shifting, 64

DF glides
general discussion, 140–141
nine minute workouts, 275–276
in 13-week program, 228

diet, 290, 294

difficulty level of exercise, adjusting, 295–296

dips, 133–134

dirty dogs
    general discussion, 49
    in 13-week program
    in active recovery,
        238–239, 244
    in Block 1 of, 206–207
    in Block 2 of, 218
    in Block 3 of, 230
disability, avoiding, 25
dive bombers
    general discussion, 140
    starfish, 179–181
    in 13-week program, 212–213
doctors, consulting before
    beginning exercise
    regimen, 64
dynamic squats, 105–106

E

elastic bands, 17
elderly, mobility in, 258, 264
equipment for calisthenics,
    14–18
excuses, facing down, 39–40
exercise machines, 295
exercise terms, 27–28

F

fat
    burning more, 10–11, 33–34
    myths about muscles and, 294
feet, parallel, 27
filming exercises, 17
fitness
    developmental movements,
        23–25
    function and, 19–20
    living pain free, 26–27
    locomotion, 20–21
    performance leads to
        efficiency, 28–30
    performance pyramid, 25

during pregnancy, 251–254
    strengthening structure of
        body, 21–23
flexibility, 14
floor exercises
    back lying exercises
        dead bugs, 45–46
        glute hip-ups, 46–47
        up and overs, 47–48
        windshield wipers, 48–49
    for children, 266
    coordination, improving, 44
    crawling exercises
        dirty dogs, 49
        hip circles, 50
        pointers, 51
        straight wide legs, 52
    front lying exercises
        hip twists, 53–54
        moose antlers, 54
        twists and reaches, 55
        Y-cuffs, 55–57
    hip, spine, and shoulder
        functions, improving, 44
    limited mobility, working out
        with, 256–257
    overview, 43
    posture, improving, 44
    side lying exercises
        hip drops, 57–58
        moon walks, 58–59
        side crunches, 59–60
        side leg lifts, 60–61
    suggested weekly regimen
        for, 45
    warm ups, 195
flows, 189–190
force absorption, 24
forearms, strength training for.
    See pulling exercises
form, focusing on, 35
Friday workouts, 13-week
    program

active recovery week, 244–245
Block 1 (weeks 1-4), 208–210
Block 2 (weeks 5-8), 220–222
Block 3 (weeks 9-12), 232–234
front lunges, 108
front lying exercises
    hip twists, 53–54
    moose antlers, 54
    in 13-week program
        in active recovery, 240–242,
            245–247
        in Block 1 of, 210–211
        in Block 2 of, 222–223
        in Block 3 of, 234–236
    twists and reaches, 55
    Y-cuffs, 55–57
full body training splits,
    191–192, 194
functional fitness, 19–20
future benefits of calisthenics,
    266–267

G

gate swings, 121–122
gear for calisthenics, 14–18
getting up and down from floor,
    with limited mobility, 259
glute hip-ups
    general discussion, 46–47
    in 13-week program
        in active recovery, 237,
            242–243
        in Block 1 of, 201, 202, 203
        in Block 2 of, 215, 216
        in Block 3 of, 227
glutes, nine minute workout for,
    282–283
goals
    adapting workouts for,
        193–195
    choosing type of workout
        circuit training, 189
        flows, 189–190

goals *(continued)*
  ladders, 187–188
  overview, 185–186
  sets across, 186
  speed sets, 188
  supersets, 186–187
  timed sets, 188
  clarifying, 31–35
  excuses, facing down, 39–40
  focusing on form not
    weights, 35
  injury, avoiding, 195–196
  motivation, finding and
    keeping, 36–38
  overcoming obstacles, 38–39
  starting small, 36
  training splits, 191–193
  true measure of merit, 36
gym workouts versus
  calisthenics, 8–10

H

hanging leg lifts, 79, 80
health, prioritizing, 38
high kicks, 170–171
high knee marches, 124
high knee runs, 124–125
high knee skips, 125–126
hip circles
  general discussion, 50
  nine minute workouts, 284
  in 13-week program
    in active recovery, 239, 244
    in Block 1 of, 207
    in Block 2 of, 219
    in Block 3 of, 231
hip drops
  general discussion, 57–58
  starfish, 177, 178
hip function
  coordinated hip and shoulder
    exercises

kneeling to standing
  exercises, 67
lying to kneeling exercises,
  65–66
from lying to stork stance
  exercises, 68–69
rolling exercises, 64–65
improving, 44
pain, lessening, 26–27
hip hinging exercises
  Bulgarian split squats, 104–105
  deadlifts, 92–93
  deadlifts to squats, 100–102
  dynamic squats, 105–106
  narrow squats, 96–97
  nine minute workouts, 273,
    278–281
  one-legged deadlifts, 93–94
  one-legged Romanian
    deadlifts, 95–96
  one-legged squats, 102–103
  overhead squats, 99
  Romanian deadlifts, 94–95
  rules for, 92
  squat thrusts, 103–104
  squats to deadlifts, 100
  T-arm squats, 98
  wide squats, 97
hip swirls, 159–160
hip twists
  general discussion, 53–54
  in 13-week program
    in active recovery, 240, 246
    in Block 1 of, 210
    in Block 2 of, 222
    in Block 3 of, 234
home, body as, 18
household items, using as gear,
  14–17

I

icons, used in book, 3
ideal alignment, maintaining, 128

inch worm exercises
  bloomers, 163–165
  deep squats, 165
  kneeling switches, 168–169
  overview, 163
  vertical twists, 165–167
independent workouts, 37
injuries
  avoiding, 11, 26, 195–196
  children's resistance to,
    267–268
  dealing with, 38
  during pregnancy, 252
inline pulling exercises
  assisted and negative pull-ups,
    154–155
  overview, 150
  pull-ups, 151–153
inline pushing exercises
  bear crawls, 141–142
  DF glides, 140–141
  dive bombers, 140
  military presses, 138–139
  overview, 137
intensity, adjusting,
  193–194, 253
Iron Mikes, 113–114
ITB kickouts, 87
ITB leg lifts, 86

J

jack knives, 84
joint alignment, ideal, 22
joint functions, 22–23, 195

K

kickouts
  general discussion, 169–170
  in 13-week program, 225,
    226, 233
knee pain, lessening, 26–27
kneeling properly, 26

About the Authors

Mark Lauren (Tampa Bay, FL) is an internationally recognized expert in body-weight training. For 15 years, Mark was a military physical-training specialist. He is also a triathlete and a champion Thai boxer, and he enjoys being a personal trainer to civilian men and women of all fitness levels. He is the author of many books, including the internationally popular *You Are Your Own Gym, Body By You, Body Fuel, and Strong and Lean*. Visit his website at https://marklauren.com.

Joshua Clark is the author of *Heart Like Water*, a finalist for the National Book Critics Circle award, and *Leopard*, a semi-finalist for the Oscars screenplay fellow-ship. Clark received an Economics degree from Yale University, has served as a correspondent for National Public Radio, and was an editor for *SCAT Magazine*. His books have been translated into 11 languages and counting. With Mark Lauren, he co-authored the international bestseller fitness books *You Are Your Own Gym, Body By You, and Strong and Lean*. He is the president of the non-profit foundation Lifeline USA Ukraine.

Authors' Acknowledgments

Behind every successful book there is a dedicated team of individuals who self-lessly contribute their time, energy, and expertise.

With unwavering dedication, unparalleled expertise, and a steadfast belief in our work, Steve Ross has been a strong driving force behind our most successful literary creations, to include *You Are Your Own Gym, Strong and Lean*, and now *Calisthenics For Dummies*. This book would not have come into existence without his tireless efforts and empathetic mentorship. Thank you!

Mark is also immensely grateful for the ongoing support of Lea Badenhoop. Her organizational skills, attention to detail, and absolute dedication are invaluable to his organization's success.

Lastly, we would like to thank the Dummies team for this rare opportunity. It is an honor to become one of your authors and subject matter experts. The relentless drive and firm guidance of our editors Kezia Endsley and Jennifer Yee did not go unnoticed, and it is in the end greatly appreciated! Thank you.

Publisher's Acknowledgments

Acquisitions Editor: Jennifer Yee

Managing Editor:
Murari Mukundan/Kristie Pyles

Project Editor: Kezia Endsley

Technical Editor: Lou Schuler

Production Editor: Pradesh Kumar

Cover Image: © skynesher/Getty Images